THE GREAT BOOK OF
HEMP

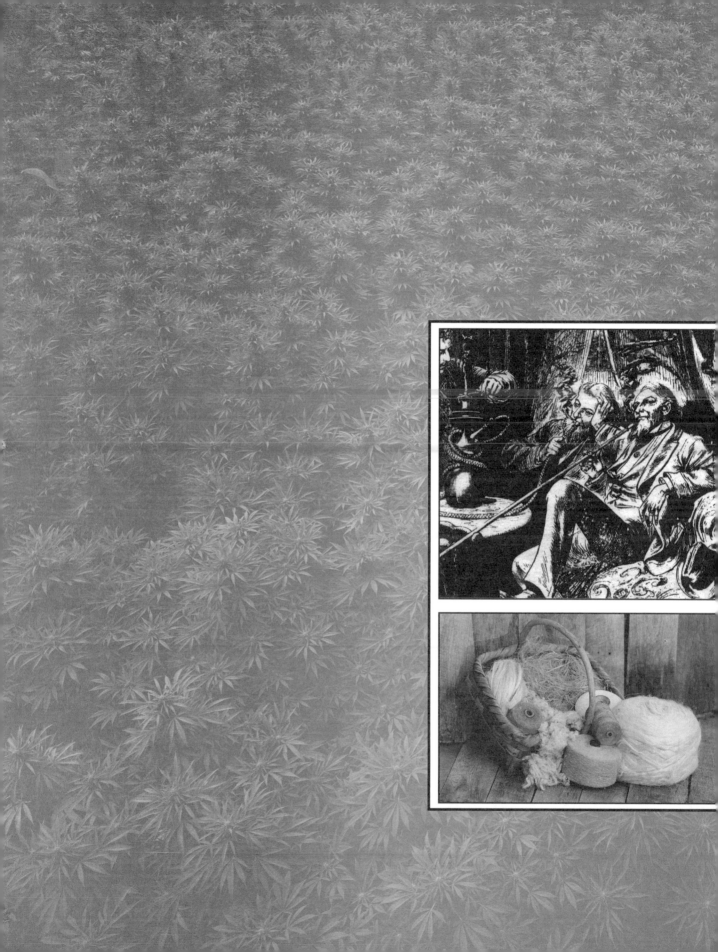

THE GREAT BOOK OF
HEMP

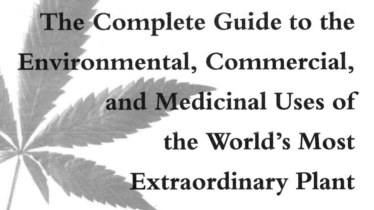

The Complete Guide to the Environmental, Commercial, and Medicinal Uses of the World's Most Extraordinary Plant

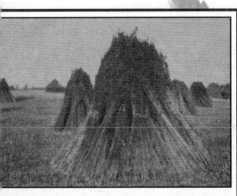

ROWAN ROBINSON

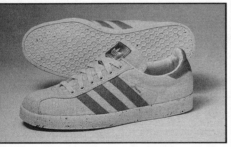

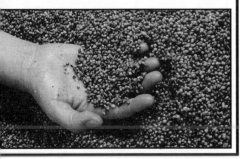

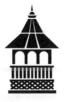

Park Street Press
Rochester, Vermont

Park Street Press
One Park Street
Rochester, Vermont 05767
Web Site: http://www.gotoit.com

LIBRARY OF CONGRESS CATALOGING-IN-PUBLICATION DATA

Robinson, Rowan.
The great book of hemp : the complete guide to the environmental, commercial, and
medicinal uses of the world's most extraordinary plant / Rowan Robinson.
p.   cm.
Includes bibliographical references and index.
ISBN 0-89281-541-8
1. Cannabis.   2. Cannabis—United States.   3. Hemp.   4. Hemp—United States.   I. Title.
HV5822.C3R65   1995
615'.7827–dc20   95–33699
CIP

Printed and bound in the United States.

10 9 8 7 6 5 4 3 2

Text design and layout by Virginia L. Scott

This book was typeset in Stone Sans with Craw Modern as the display typeface

On the cover: Declaration of Independence courtesy of Superstock;
other photographs courtesy of Andre Grossman

Photographs on pages i, ii, and iii: marijuana leaf and hemp field background
by Andre Grossman; hemp twine and cord courtesy of The Ohio Hempery;
hemp stalks from USDA 1913 Yearbook; Adidas shoes courtesy of Adidas America;
photograph of hemp seeds by Mari Kane.

Photographs courtesy of Superstock on pages 21, 22, 26, 125, 131, 133, 148

Photographs courtesy of The Bettmann Archives on pages 150, 165

Park Street Press is a division of Inner Traditions International

Distributed to the book trade in Canada by Publishers Group West (PGW),
Toronto, Ontario
Distributed to the book trade in the United Kingdom by Deep Books, London
Distributed to the book trade in Australia by Millennium Books, Newtown, N.S.W.
Distributed to the book trade in New Zealand by Tandem Press, Auckland
Distributed to the book trade in South Africa by Alternative Books, Randburg

In all cases the publisher has made every effort to contact and get permission
from the artists and appropriate institutions for the images and
photographs in this book. Nevertheless if omissions or errors have occured,
we encourage you to contact Inner Traditions International.

CONTENTS

PUBLISHER'S FOREWORD

Can there be a special relationship between a plant and mankind? How is it that out of the billions of life forms on earth only an infinitesimally small number have a relationship with humanity? In the animal kingdom we have a special relationship with cows, dogs, cats, horses, and a few other animals that live close to us, with whom we share our lives and who in turn give us benefits. It would be hard to imagine living without these special and intimate relationships which have traveled with us since our earliest historic memories.

But what of the plant kingdom? Are there relationships so close and intimately tied to our own that human development as we know it could not have happened without their help? Trees give us wood to build, and cotton clothes us. Wheat, corn, and other grains feed us. Healing herbs are there to comfort us when we are sick, and numerous other plants are available to support and assist us in our human endeavor. However, there is only one plant helper used all over the world, since prehistory, that gives us food, clothing, building materials, fuel, medicine, and has the power to affect our consciousness, our imagination, and the way we see that world. That plant is hemp, *Cannabis sativa*.

Hemp appears on the world stage at the dawn of human experience. We find its seeds, rope, and cloth in the oldest tombs. In its role as healer, it is found in our earliest medical texts. We find hemp playing a key role in so many of modern history's great moments. When Gutenberg's presses started rolling, it was hemp paper that received the ink and spread the word of the Bible to an awakening Europe. When the urge to find a new world, a new way of living, gave rise to the age of discovery some 500 years ago, it was hemp that powered this urge, giving the explorers the sails and cordage needed to cross the oceans. When it came time to define this new world, its goals and aspirations, it was on hemp paper that the drafts of the United States Constitution and Declaration of Independence were written. As the young nation moved west it was hemp that covered the settlers' wagons.

Even after being outlawed, this fugitive plant has returned to help us in times of special need. During World War II when supplies of raw fiber were cut off by the Japanese, hemp was reintroduced to the U.S. farmer to support the war effort, as the U.S. Department of Agriculture proclaimed "hemp for victory." In the 1960s a movement of youth inspired by the ideals of peace and love burst on to the world stage challenging the social, economic, and religious order of the day. This movement of millions upon millions had no leaders, no ideology, no strategy for change, only a deep rooted sense of the hypocrisy

of the "establishment's materialistic world view" and a special relationship with a plant—a plant that has receptors in the human brain waiting to receive its biochemical messages. A message of respect for the earth, its plants and animals, for our bodies and the foods we eat, for cultures and people other than our own was heard and the sea of change it brought is still being played out today.

How extraordinary that hemp should once again appear, but this time in the role of environmentalist and healer. Today hemp offers us a very real and immediate solution to deforestation, the abuses of the petrochemical industry, and the destruction of our top soils as well as help in health care problems as diverse as glaucoma and A.I.D.S.

Only the arrogance of the modern mentality, worshipping at the altar of the church of progress, would reject and deny the history and virtues of hemp. Is it necessary to fear and outlaw this plant? Or are we really trying to outlaw a change in consciousness? Try as we may, a change in culture and consciousness is already happening—a change that is earth-honoring and embraces the healing, environmental, and spiritual qualities of this special relationship between hemp and humanity.

Ehud C. Sperling

ACKNOWLEDGMENTS

Even more so than most books, this project would not have been possible without the help of a number of people. Thank you to Alan Reder, Ellen Komp, and Chris Conrad for their contributions, and especially to Chris for his substantial input in the discussion of hemp's energy potential. John Birrenbach, Gero Lesor, and John McPartland provided valuable feedback on the book, and Mari Kane was a constant help. Most of all, I'd like to thank Robin Dutcher-Bayer, Mary Elder Jacobsen, Janet Jesso, Tim Jones, Wendy Pratt, Virginia Scott, Lee Wood, and the rest of the amazing staff at Inner Traditions for their dedication and belief in this book. It has been a pleasure to work with you all.

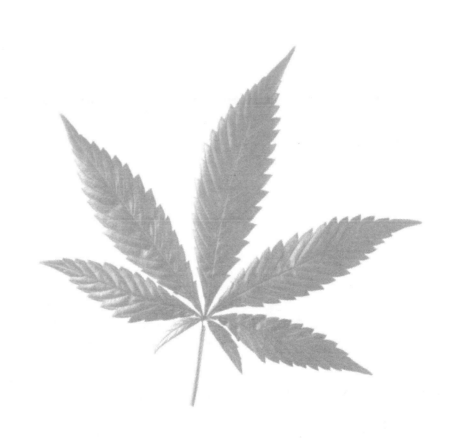

INTRODUCTION

H emp is happening. The last several years have rapidly transformed the concept of a modern industrial hemp industry from fantasy to reality. The physical presence of hemp clothing, paper, building materials, and seed-oil products has made a huge impact on our collective imagination—perhaps even more so than information about the importance of hemp in the past that was the seed of hemp's reemergence.

Since the 1930s there has been an effort to indoctrinate people with the belief that hemp is nothing more than a "devil weed with roots in hell." But when they are shown a shirt that looks like linen and told it is made from the stalk of the same plant that produces marijuana, a profound shift in awareness begins. The realization occurs that hemp is not a deadly "drug" but simply a God-given plant, one with a long and distinguished history of service to mankind.

It is significant that this awareness is blossoming while a generation is still alive that remembers the pre-1937 world when hemp was grown on the family farm, that knows the texture and flavor of an old friend when they feel it or taste it. Old-time hemp farmers and their children are still around to attest to the existence—and the value—of industrial hemp.

The resurgence of marijuana use in the late 1960s and the 1970s sparked a deluge of research on all aspects of the hemp plant. The history

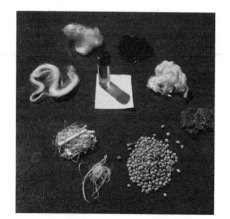

SEEDS, POWDER, PERFUME, CREAM, PAPER, AND FIBER—ALL MADE FROM HEMP. PHOTOGRAPH BY ANDRE GROSSMAN.

of hemp clothing and paper merited a chapter or two in books, largely concerned with marijuana, by Ernest Abel, Alan Haney, and Benjamin Kutscheid. By the mid-1980s researchers Gatewood Galbraith, Barry Stull, Jack Frazier, and Jack Herer were focusing their efforts on the "other" uses of the hemp plant. Government documents, newspaper accounts, and personal testimony began to unravel a vast hidden history of hemp's usefulness to mankind and the mysterious nature of government repression of the hemp plant. This hemp information soon spread to the still active pro-marijuana movement, revitalizing it with a new generation of environmental activists who were mainly concerned with ending deforestation and the use of pesticides by switching to sustainably grown hemp for paper and textiles.

It was only a matter of time before American entrepreneurs tried importing products made from hemp. In 1987 the only hemp products available in the United States were Hungarian twine, a few specialty papers such as cigarette papers, and sterilized bird seed. In 1989 a group called Business Alliance for Commerce in Hemp (BACH) uncovered and published U.S. Customs hemp import codes, which specifically

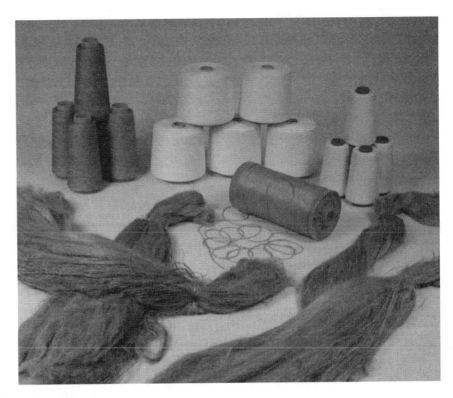

HEMP TWINE, UNCHANGED FOR MILLENIA. COURTESY OF INSTITUT FÜR ANGEWANDTE FORSCHUNG.

exclude the stalk and sterilized seed, making these imported items legal for trade. By the summer of 1989, the organization had produced several pieces of literature encouraging hemp entrepreneurs to get started in business and giving them the tools to do it. Education was a major part of early marketing strategy, and BACH fliers like "The Many Uses of Hemp" were spread far and wide by its representatives. The focus was on the environmental and economic advantages of hemp for fiber, food, and fuel.

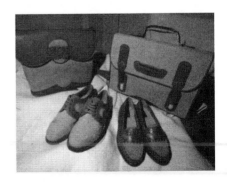

THE SOPHISTICATED SIDE OF HEMP. PHOTOGRAPH BY ANDRE GROSSMAN.

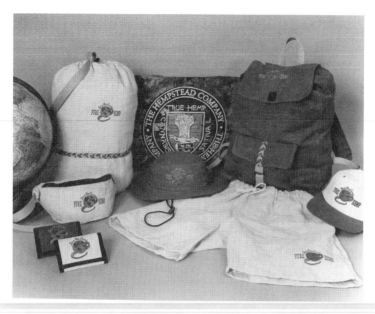

THE BEGINNING OF THE HEMP RENAISSANCE. PHOTOGRAPH BY JEFF EICHEN.

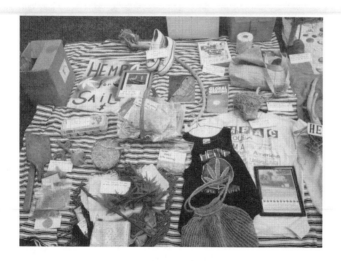

RICHARD DAVIS'S TRAVELING HEMP MUSEUM.
PHOTOGRAPH BY BILL BRIDGES.

A few items like hemp twine and sterile seeds were often shown or sold at community advocacy tables. Thousands of hand-crocheted bracelets, hats, and bags soon appeared. House of Hemp in Portland, Oregon, contracted to import 100 percent hemp canvas from China, to sell for upholstery fabric, carpet backing, and the like. Entrepreneurs quickly bought the fabric and began stitching hats, bags, and clothing from the sturdy cloth. Singer Willie Nelson got into the act in 1991, licensing his signature for a hemp-cotton shirt and speaking about hemp at his Farm Aid concerts. Tree-Free EcoPaper brought the first loads of hemp and cereal straw paper to the United States in September 1992.

A healthy hemp-rally circuit gave hemp entrepreneurs a start, selling their wares while distributing literature at outdoor rallies across the country. The American Hemp Council, a community group started in Los Angeles, held quarterly rallies that drew up to ten thousand starting in late 1991, funding their efforts with sales of hemp-seed pancakes. This new breed of hemp rally joined forces with established pro-marijuana rallies like the Michigan Hash Bash, Madison Harvest Fest, and the Atlanta Pot Festival, and hemp vendors soon branched out to environmental fairs, craft fairs, and music festivals.

BACH had displays at sixty-seven Earth Day events in 1991.

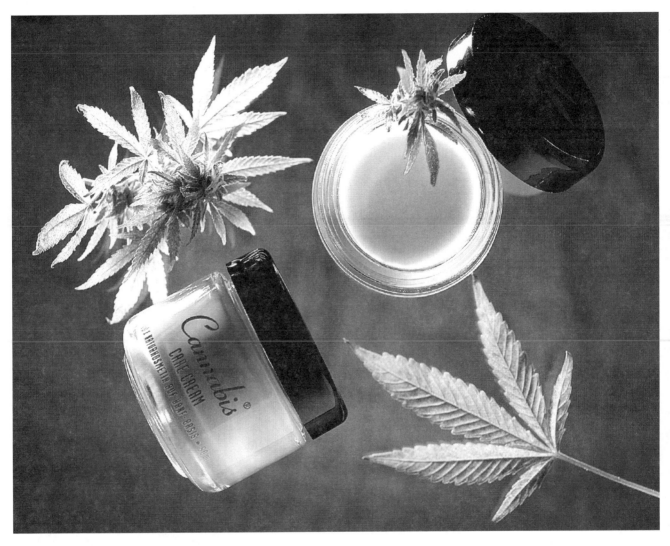

SKIN CREAM FROM HEMP-SEED OIL—ONE OF THE HEALTHIEST OILS KNOWN TO MAN.
PHOTOGRAPH COURTESY OF DUPETIT NATURAL.

In 1992 more than twenty hemp companies were in business. Hemp's success, quality, and ecological merits began to catch the attention of experienced manufacturers, designers, and retailers, and the "marijuana connection" diminished as a new professionalism emerged. *HempWorld*, an industry trade journal, made its debut in December 1993. Founder Mari Kane vowed the publication would be a "capitalist tool," devoid of pro-marijuana rhetoric. "After all the ideological and economic excesses of the past 12 years, the public is desperate for something solid to believe in," Kane announced in her opening editor's statement. "Hemp is fresh, hip yet earthy, environmentally friendly, more durable than cotton, and it has enough mystique to arouse the curiosity of the most jaded cynic." The forty-two-page bimonthly publication has been an important networking and legitimizing tool for the fledgling industry.

In late 1994 forty companies met in Arizona to form the Hemp Industries Association to promote hemp, set product standards, and bring hemp farming back to America. The organization is similar to trade organizations promoting cotton, wool, and linen, and it has recently opened an office in the heart of New York's fashion world, at 42nd Street and Broadway.

Today there are more than three hundred hemp companies in the United States alone, importing, manufacturing, distributing, or retailing hundreds of products, from shoes and sandals to hemp-silk lingerie; hemp-seed oil shampoos, lip balms, and salves; handmade papers and copier-quality reams. By conservative estimates, hemp is a $15 million business domestically, and $50 million worldwide. The Real

Goods catalog carries hemp, as do Patagonia and Sundance. Hemp is gaining more respectability every day, and big-time companies and designers like Converse, Ralph Lauren, and Calvin Klein are starting to dip their toes into hempen waters. Hemp retail stores have opened their doors in cities throughout the United States, Europe, Canada, and Australia. Many of these companies, as well as the Institute for Hemp, the Coalition for Hemp Awareness, and Hemp BC, also operate virtual stores on the Internet's worldwide web.

The United States and Germany, where growing restrictions are harshest, have nurtured the most successful hemp businesses. German interest is attributed to a strong green movement. Hemp made an impressive presence in early 1995 at Germany's Biofach, the world's largest ecological-consumer-goods trade show. A four-day conference attended by scientists and industrialists from around the world discussed breeding, harvesting, and storage techniques; processing, retting, and finishing for paper pulp and fiber; hemp seeds for human nutrition, cosmetics, and detergents; building materials, fuel, and medical applications; and legal issues. Forty different hemp companies from nine countries participated

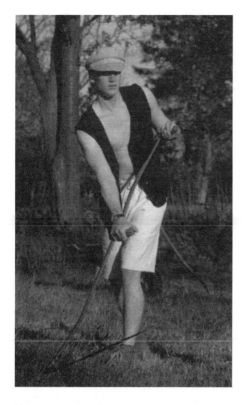 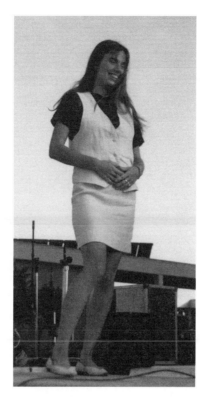

HEMP FASHIONS. LEFT PHOTOGRAPH COURTESY OF CANNABIS IN BERLIN. RIGHT PHOTOGRAPH BY BILL BRIDGES.

on the trade-show floor. Some of the newer products seen were hemp particle board pressed and molded into bowls and dash-boards, fiber-matting material similar to fiberglass for use as pad-ding or insulation, hemp laces, hemp-oil detergent and cosmetics, and plastic from hemp cellulose to be marketed to skateboard manu-facturers. At Biofach, American hemp entrepreneurs finally achieved a longed-for legitimacy as eco-businesses.

Hemp Textiles

You may be wearing more hemp than you know. Designer Ralph Lauren recently revealed that he has been secretly using hemp fiber in his clothing lines since 1984. In a June 1995 article titled "World's Oldest Fabric Is Now Its Newest," the *New York Times* "outed" Lauren and interviewed Calvin Klein, who said, "I believe that hemp is going to be the fiber of choice in both the home furnishings and fashion

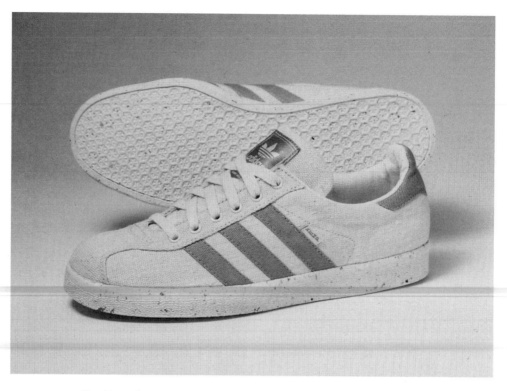

THE HEMP SHOE, MADE BY ADIDAS. BOTH THE UPPER AND THE LACES ARE MADE WITH HEMP CANVAS. COURTESY OF ADIDAS AMERICA.

industries." Hemp linen was featured in duvet covers, decorative pillows, and pillow shams in the fall 1995 C. K. Home Collection. Klein hinted that hemp would soon make an appearance in his clothing lines as well.

Hemp has been a utilitarian fabric for centuries, and it was natural that hemp clothing would be among the first products to hit today's ecology-conscious fashion market. In only a few years, hemp fashions have skyrocketed from obscurity to notoriety. Many magazines have shown hemp fashions on their pages and *Rolling Stone* listed hemp in its 1993 "hot" list. MTV, CNN, Fox, CBS, and ABC have all focused on the new looks.

Hemp isn't just a trendy new fabric, however. It's a classic. Hemp fiber bundles are up to fifteen feet long, while cotton fibers are a mere three-quarters of an inch, which reportedly gives hemp eight times the tensile strength and four times the durability of cotton. Hemp is machine washable and

■■■

Cannabis is the original and only "true Hemp." In the past century especially, several other fiber plants have assumed the generic name "hemp": Manila hemp is also known as abaca *(Musa textilis);* Sisal hemp is henequen *(Agave fourcroydes* L.*);* New Zealand hemp is *Phormium tenax;* Mauritius hemp is *Furcraea foetida;* deccan hemp is *Hibiscus cannabinus;* and Sunn hemp is *Crotolaria juncea.* Jute *(Corchorus capsularis* L.*)* also is known as Indian hemp—not to be confused with *Cannabis indica,* which *used* to be called Indian hemp.[2]

Foreign-milled hemp-cotton blends abound in hemp fashions today. Though the blend sacrifices strength (in comparison to that offered by a pure hemp product), it offers the advantages of more softness, better moisture wicking, and a lower price. Several companies have begun using hemp-cotton twills as well as 100 percent hemp denim in jeans. Hemp-silk blends have recently been introduced that combine softness and strength.

Pure, 100 percent hemp is nonetheless the way hemp makes its appearance in designs today, usually in its natural off-white color (similar to organic cotton). Chinese linen and the stiffer and darker Hungarian and Russian hemp fabrics abound in men's, women's, and children's wear, as well as in accessories like hats, bags,

and shoes. English hemp, some of it mixed with recycled wool or recycled cotton from blue jeans, is also appearing. One enterprising company, Pan World Traders, traveled to Transylvania to purchase an-

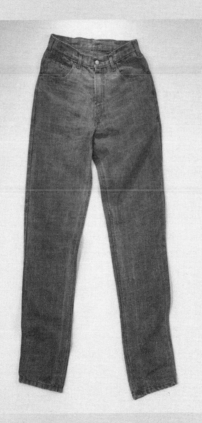

100% HEMP JEANS. PHOTOGRAPH BY ANDRE GROSSMAN.

tique hemp linens one household at a time. They hand-dyed and stitched the fine fabric into caps, packs, neckties, and handkerchiefs.

The hemp textile industry encompasses manufacturers of all sizes, from small cooperatives stitching a few items to large factories,

foreign and domestic, turning out thousands of garments daily. For example, Headcase turns out one thousand hemp baseball caps a day. Most items are still sold by catalog or in hemp specialty stores, but more and more they are seen as just another fabric in boutiques and department stores. This move beyond a niche market is critical for clothing. The vast majority of consumers buy their clothing in stores where they can try the items on and compare prices. Hemp's higher price can be offset by its superior quality and styling and by marketing it as an environmental option.

Established enviro-wear companies are starting to make use of hemp. Used Rubber, a San Francisco company making bags, belts, and accessories from recycled rubber, added hemp as the first fabric in their line when they discovered its ecological advantages. Deja Shoe, recipient of the United Nations' Fashion Industry and the Environment Award for their recycled-products shoes, introduced a line of hemp-fabric footwear in early 1995. Bob Farentinos, former vice-president of environmental affairs at Deja, said his technical people call hemp fabric "bullet-proof." "Hemp fulfills our mission of using sustainably harvested plant material in our shoes," he said. "It's hard to beat hemp for all of its advantages."

■■■

dryable. Although it will wrinkle like a natural linen, it also breathes like one. Hemp has a natural luster and takes dyes beautifully, due to its superior absorbency.

Many people imagine hemp looks like burlap. In fact, the strength and coarseness of a fabric depends on how the fiber is spun and woven. Hemp, like flax and other fibers, can be woven in many grades, from canvas to fine linen. With proper processing, hemp can be made softer than cotton. It is also more absorbent, making it an excellent choice for towels, diapers, and baby clothing. Upholstery fabric, table linens, casual clothing, and high-quality linen wear are all potential markets for hemp.

Industrial textiles and apparel now account for 59 percent of the United States' imports and 21 percent of the United States' trade deficit. The machinery no longer exists to spin long fibers like flax and hemp, but hemp can be extruded into rayon or shortened, like cotton, for existing machinery. Retooling would enable more types of weaves that take advantage of the longer fiber length hemp offers, and create an economic opportunity that should not be underestimated. During World War II, the cost of retooling for hemp was paid in just five years with rentals and profits.[1]

Because of limited cultivation, hemp fabrics on the market today are somewhat scarce. That situation is rapidly improving. Owen Sercus, a professor of fabric finishing at New York's Fashion Institute of Technology, has been working with the Hemp Industries Association to establish testing and certification standards for hemp in the United States. Through his workshops, hemp entrepreneurs have learned to demand greater authenticity, quality, and consistency from their sources. A "True Hemp" certification label has been developed to assure customers that what they are getting is in fact high-quality *Cannabis sativa* L.

Hemp Paper

Hemp's biggest contribution to the world's economy and ecology could well be as part of a return to plant-based papers. Half of all trees cut down are used to make paper, and deforestation is a serious environmental crisis, weakening our ecosystems, topsoil, and watersheds, as well as increasing the greenhouse effect. Trees have been used for paper only since the mid-1800s. Before then, paper was made from cloth rags and annual crops like papyrus and hemp. In addition, an estimated 1.5 billion tons of agricultural waste is produced annually, and this is waste that could be turned into paper, especially with the addition of a long fiber like hemp. With paper prices soaring and shortages abounding, now is the time to look at what are currently called "alternative" sources of paper pulp.

Hemp-paper prices in the 1990s have been quite a bit higher than tree-pulp paper, but comparable to other annual fiber papers like cotton. The major difficulty is that only a handful of domestic mills can handle the fiber. With investment capital for development costs and cooperation with the nonwood paper industry, hemp-paper suppliers are working to bring the cost of their product down and the quality up.

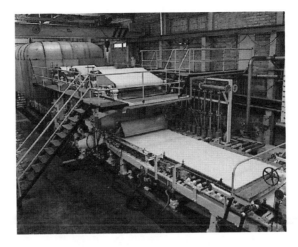

LIVING TREE PAPER COMPANY'S HEMP PAPER MILL.

Home-grown Housing and Industrial Products

The cannabis hemp stalk is a prolific and sustainable source of excellent building materials and manufactured goods. It is possible to build, for example, a car body or a house almost entirely out of hemp, and then use hemp-seed oil products to paint and seal the finished

■■■

One of the promising hemp companies of the 1990s is Living Tree Paper Company in Eugene, Oregon, which markets Tradition Bond™, an American made tree-free hemp paper, the first hemp content paper to be milled (starting in early 1995) in the U.S. on a commercial basis. By using a blend of hemp, esparto-grass, agricultural by-products, and postconsumer waste, Living Tree offers a paper which does not use trees, relieves already overburdened landfills, and is significantly better for the environment than recycled paper, which usually contains less than 10 percent postconsumer waste.

EPA guidelines for labeling a product recycled call for using only 10 percent "reclaimed" preconsumer waste such as mill broke, the scraps of paper that are trimmed off in the mill and reused anyway as standard operating procedure. Thus, a "recycled" paper may be made of 90 percent virgin-wood pulp. Postconsumer waste includes newspapers, magazines, cardboard, and so forth, which require de-inking before they can be repulped; this filthy process actually produces more pollution than does the manufacture of virgin paper. Wood pulp produces one-third paper and two-thirds waste. One hundred tons of paper made from virgin-wood fiber produces about five tons of sludge, some of which can be used as fertilizer. One hundred tons of paper made from postconsumer waste generates about forty tons of toxic sludge, which must be disposed of.

■■■

■■■

The pioneering C&S Specialty Builders Supply in Harrisburg, Oregon, produces superlative composite fiberboard from hemp. The medium density fiber (MDF) composite boards are 250 percent stronger than wood MDF composite board, and 300 percent more elastic. The product was developed in conjunction with Washington State University's wood-research center.

After a lengthy and detailed survey of the plant kingdom and extensive historical research about the uses of plants in civilization, C&S Specialty Builders Supply concluded that the absolute best alternative to wood in construction products is hemp. In fact, they believe hemp has the potential to be vastly superior to wood for everything from lumber to plywood to particle board. Additionally they think hemp cores have great potential to make glues for composite construction products.

"I think that if we don't do it [grow hemp] there is a good chance that in ten years there will be no forests left on the temperate region of the Earth," says company co-founder David Seber. "The overriding issue about the forests is not about trees, and it's not even about wood, it's about fiber, and how our culture uses fiber. . . . Not only do we have the solution to the forests, we have the only really viable concept of what sustainability is about. We're saying you don't take a two-hundred- to five-hundred-year-old plant—namely a tree—to make a house that lasts fifty years. You take a plant that takes one hundred days to grow to make a house that lasts fifty years. That gives you sustainability." Seber's partner, William Conde, adds, "The way to fix the forest is to use advanced composites from annual fibers like hemp. Anything you can make out of a tree you can make out of hemp. We can leave the forest alone and everyone can go back to work."

■■■

products and power the car.

The technology exists to switch to hemp composites or to add hemp to current processes without retooling. The challenge: to grow the fifteen hundred tons per day of raw material.

In general, the longer the fiber used, the stronger the end product is in relation to its weight. A cannabis plant can top fifteen feet, with its bark fiber bundles running virtually this entire length. That gives hemp bast exceptional strength when combined with resin binders to manufacture high-density composite materials. The Ford Motor Company investigated the possibility of using hemp in cars in 1929, and sent officials to visit the successful hemp farm of Albert Fraleigh in Alberta, Canada, before cultivating a two hundred acre crop. In the December 1941 issue of *Popular Mechanics* Henry Ford proudly displayed, after twelve years of research, the first automobile "grown from the soil" with a plastic body made from 70 percent hemp, wheat straw, and sisal with 30 percent hemp resin binder. The only steel in the car body was its welded tubular frame. The vehicle weighed a third less than its steel counterparts but demonstrated ten times the impact strength.

Medium density fiber (MDF) is a cellulosic composite comparable in strength to the wood of trees. It is used for building, cabinetry, furniture, and other carpentry and woodworking applications. Prototype hemp MDF boards surpassed their tree-based counterparts. One Dutch company grows its own hemp and is beginning to produce composite boards for housing as well as items like salad bowls and wall clocks.

Isochanvre, a French company, has already built about 250 hemp houses. It uses a patented, non-toxic method to process stalk into insulation materials and a light-weight substitute for concrete. Pulp used for its insulation is treated with a fire retardant and used either loose or still in the bag to fill and insulate spaces within walls and ceilings. The building material uses hemp chips coated with a mineral binder that is mixed with water and lime and can be cast in molds or applied with a trough. The organic material calcifies and hardens into a stable mass that is insulative of both sound and temperature. The fossilized hemp stalk retains some flexibility and when dry only weighs one-seventh as much as conventional concrete. One hectare of hemp produces about sixty cubic meters of Isochanvre—enough to build and insulate a 135-square-meter (1300-square-foot) house. Construction material now costs $215.50 per cubic meter and insulation $263.48. That's about $14,000 for the house. The company could bring down the cost of the product by growing or contracting their own hemp, but the federal monopoly on hemp farming prevents it.

Farther north, in Germany, where no hemp farming is

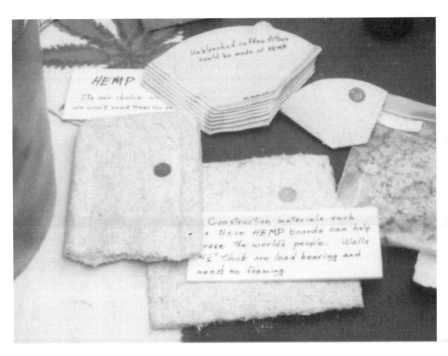

THE ORIGINAL PAPER SOURCE RETURNS. PHOTOGRAPH BY BILL BRIDGES.

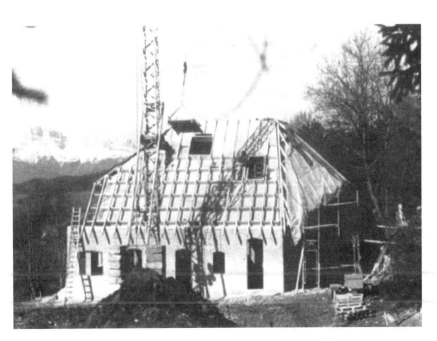

AN ISOCHANVRE HOUSE IN FRANCE. PHOTOGRAPH COURTESY OF *HEMPWORLD*.

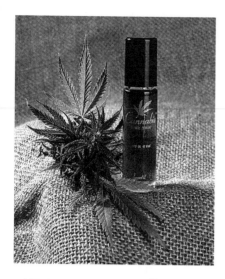

HEMP-SEED OIL PERFUME. COURTESY OF
DUPETIT NATURAL.

allowed, imported stalks are carbon-treated, packed into place, and used for loose underfloors. The bituminized material is slightly sticky and compresses to fit the contours of the lower surface. It creates an insulated and level surface for finishing the floor.

The full potential to combine hemp stalks with extrusion technology to make plastics remains largely unexplored. Greenhouse, a company based in Frankfurt, Germany, takes the finer particles of hemp pulp to make a rigid plastic-like compound that is biodegradable. The material breaks back down into hemicellulose through exposure to water. The company plans to add a good sealant and manufacture cannabis skateboards. One viable source for such a sealant is the hemp-seed oil, which can be polymerized or

made into polyurethane for a wide variety of finishes. Field-operating units are also capable of using the oil for plasticized products from foam rubber to polyconcrete—twice as strong as conventional concrete but slightly flexible. Plastic plumbing is another possibility. Can hemp fiber optics be far behind?

Seed-Oil Products

Yet another usable and potentially profitable component of the hemp plant is its seed. Before the Marihuana Tax Act of 1937, hemp-seed oil was used as a lamp oil, in paints as a drying oil, and as a varnish for wood. Printing inks were another use. At least one publisher has printed with a hemp-soy ink on hemp paper. The oil makes an excellent emollient for skin and hair, opening up the personal-care products industry to hemp-seed massage oil, salves, lip balms, body creme, shampoo, and creme rinse.

Health experts have been speaking for decades about the need for unsaturated fats in our diets, namely the fatty acids called linoleic (LA, or omega 6), and linolenic (LNA, or omega 3). Hemp seeds are treasure troves of these

---

■■■
The Marihuana Tax Act

The 1937 Marihuana Tax Act was the death blow to legal hemp farming in America. Rebuffed in its attempts to get hemp classified as a narcotic, the Federal Bureau of Narcotics resorted to an indirect assault on the plant. It pushed through congress a bill taxing hemp at the rate of $1.00 per ounce for industrial and medical purposes and $100.00 per ounce for other purposes. While theoretically a means of generating revenue, the bill was in reality designed to crush the hemp industry—imagine a $1.00 per ounce tax on corn or cotton during the Great Depression. The bill put many companies out of business and shifted the status of hemp from a legal domestic crop to an illegal imported one.

■■■

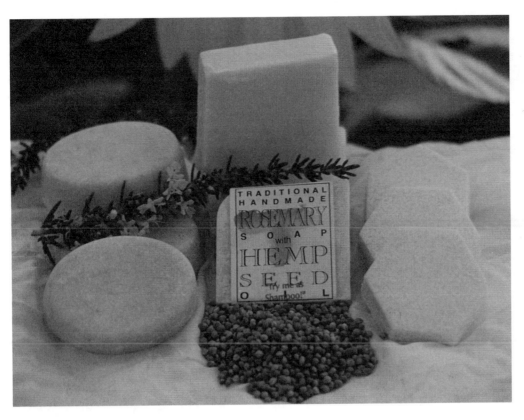

ALL-NATURAL HEMP-SEED OIL SOAP. COURTESY OF ARTHA.

nutrients. They contain at least 30 percent oil, mostly LA and LNA in the optimum three-to-one ratio. Flax oil, a comparable product, is a $6 million industry. Currently hemp-seed oil is two to three times more expensive than flax oil, but has more applications because of its superior taste, such as hemp cheese and "hempeh" burgers. Some analysts believe that, if hemp were cultivated in the United States, hemp-seed oil would be as inexpensive as corn oil.

The biggest stumbling block to marketing hemp-seed products is the government requirement to sterilize the seeds. This lessens their freshness and nutritional content. Furthermore, all imported nuts and seeds must be fumigated with methyl bromide, which is not popular with environmentally conscious health-food consumers. No traces have been found to date on imported seed because the chemical is extremely volatile, but at best it is an ozone-depleter. Some companies have begun pressing oil from unsterilized seed in Chile,

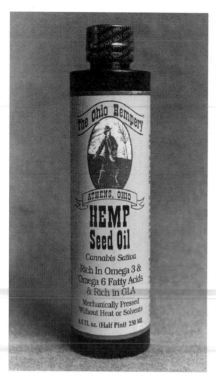

NUTRITIOUS HEMP-SEED OIL.
COURTESY OF OHIO HEMPERY.

but the cost of refrigerated transportation is just as high as the cost to domestically press the oil.

Hemp's Future

The products on the market today are but a small demonstration of the potential of hemp's usefulness for paper, fiber, food, fuel, and countless other products. Hemp is recommended for reclaiming deforested, marginal, and heavy-metal–contaminated lands, and the coming century will doubtless see a huge need for this kind of reclamation. Since hemp was suppressed just at the time when machinery would have taken hemp into the industrial age, there has never been the opportunity to take advantage of hemp as a natural resource in modern times.

Although the grassroots entrepreneurs who started the hemp revival recognize the need for involvement from larger companies to achieve the ultimate goal of domestic cultivation, they express hope that the "little guys" whose profits fund activist and education activities won't be swallowed up by corporate interests. They envision hemp as part of a move toward a more sustainable, decentralized, farm-based economy that excludes the kind of dehumanizing

and wasteful monopolization of industries past. Of course, these goals cannot be achieved without establishing localized cultivation.

Some within the industry have been critical of the "fad" hemp products that are on the market. They worry that the focus on hemp fashions instead of on more urgently needed commodities like paper and building products creates a risk that the industry will simply be a flash in the pan. Others have been critical of some members of the U.S. hemp industry for mixing hemp with the marijuana-legalization issue. Many of the products on the market feature a "hemp" leaf that most people associate with marijuana. The controversy surrounding the plant has actually worked to the hemp industry's advantage in generating publicity about its products. Network TV may not carry stories about flax or cotton, but hemp is a hot news item. Still, the contention rises that continuing to link the issues slows progress toward restoring industrial hemp.

Most hemp activists' overwhelming interest is in ecological issues, and they're tired of being accused of advancing hemp simply so they can "get stoned." With the United States in such urgent need of drug-law reform, however, it is difficult not to speak out about the injustice of marijuana laws, particularly in light of the mounting evidence for industrial-conspiracy theories along with information about marijuana's role in medicine and spirituality. More urgent, perhaps, is the economic argument. With prisons becoming the nation's number-one growth industry, the resources to develop clean, green technologies likely won't be found until the end of the War on Drugs. Furthermore, it is the drug-enforcement bureaucracy that is, time after time, mixing the issues. Although marijuana and hemp are one and the same species, they are quite different in character when bred for industrial versus medical or social consumption. With a better understanding of mankind's relationship with plant hallucinogens will come the tolerant and reasoned atmosphere under which a hemp industry will flourish.

While the European Economic Community, Canada, China, and the former Soviet Union develop hemp-seed lines and new technologies and markets, U.S. policymakers continue to feed the political pork barrel of "zero tolerance." Nevertheless, the coalition for industrial hemp is getting stronger every day, encompassing farmers, financiers, and multinational industrialists, as well as enthusiastic young entrepreneurs. The U.S. Department of Agriculture developed hybrid seed lines in the early 1900s that, by their reports, produce greater yields than hemp grown anywhere else. It is only a matter of time before the U.S. also will take advantage of hemp, once described by the framers of the U.S. Constitution, Gouverneur Morris and Thomas Jefferson, as being "of first necessity . . . to the wealth and protection of the country."

Ellen Komp and Chris Conrad

1

THE ENVIRONMENT AND HEMP HUSBANDRY

S ay you are the United States government. You are presiding over a runaway technological freight train heading for the brink of environmental collapse. More and more of your scientists are sounding the alarm: heavy reliance on fossil fuels is causing soaring pollution levels and increasingly acidic rain. Your forests are disappearing at an alarming rate to serve the housing and paper industries, leaving behind vast tracts of eroding soil. Farmlands that have not eroded are so overused and contaminated with pesticides and insecticides from cotton and other crops that farmers must add as much as forty times the fertilizer they did a century ago to get the same yield. And the runoff from this soil is contributing to the degradation of your water supply.

You're in trouble, United States.

What you need is a new industry, one that can fill the needs now met by fossil fuels and virgin timber; one that can be worked

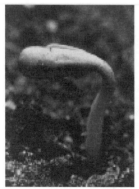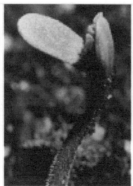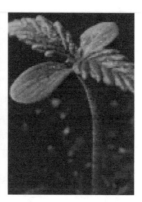

A HEMP PLANT IS BORN. PHOTOGRAPHS BY RICHARDSON, WOODS, AND BOGART.

sustainably without polluting soil, air, or water; one that is self-sufficient and local, neither exploiting nor dependent on foreign countries. This industry would need to employ those citizens previously employed by the petrochemical, timber, and cotton industries.

Say a plant is identified that miraculously fits this bill—and even *cleans* contaminated soil. Would you quickly put programs into place to encourage the cultivation of the plant and its attendant industry?

That's not what the U.S. government did. Instead, they made the plant illegal.

The plant in the above situation, of course, is hemp. *Cannabis sativa*. And the situation does not apply to the United States alone. Every industrialized nation faces environmental degradation and has potential salvation at hand in the form of this plant. All hemp is illegal in the United States, even hemp bred to not produce significant amounts of THC, the psychoactive chemical in hemp. In the words of environmental activist Andy Kerr, "Your lungs will fail before your brain attains any high from smoking industrial hemp."[1] Why the U.S. fails to distinguish between industrial hemp and psychoactive marijuana, when so many other countries are already

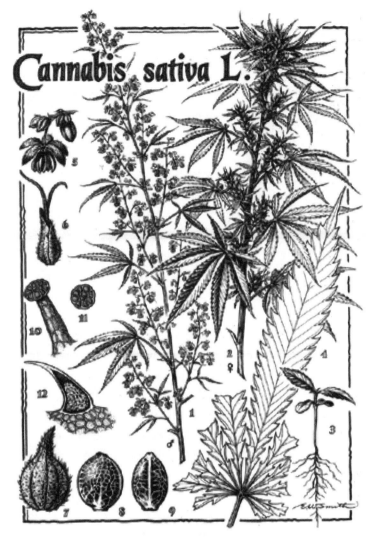

(1) TOP OF MALE PLANT, IN FLOWER; (2) TOP OF FEMALE PLANT, IN FRUIT; (3) SEEDLING; (4) LEAFLET FROM LARGE, 11-PARTED LEAF; (5) PORTION OF A STAMINATE INFLORESCENCE, WITH BUDS AND MATURE MALE FLOWER; (6) FEMALE FLOWERS, WITH STIGMAS PROTRUDING FROM HAIRY BRACT; (7) FRUIT ENCLOSED IN PERSISTENT HAIRY BRACT; (8) FRUIT, LATERAL VIEW; (9) FRUIT, END VIEW; (10) GLANDULAR HAIR WITH MULTI-CELLULAR STALK; (11) GLANDULAR HAIR WITH SHORT, ONE-CELLED INVISIBLE STALK; (12) NON-GLANDULAR HAIR CONTAINING A CYSTOLITH. ILLUSTRATION BY E. W. SMITH.

growing hemp, is a provocative question. But if one subscribes to the "trickle up" theory of governmental enlightenment—that not until nearly everyone in the coun-

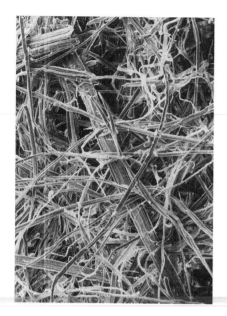

HEMP FIBER, AS SEEN THROUGH AN ELECTRON MICROSCOPE. COURTESY OF INSTITUT FÜR ANGEWANDTE FORSCHUNG.

try understands an issue will government begin to catch on—then it becomes clear that the first step must be dissemination of information. What's so wonderful about hemp? Glad you asked.

Hemp: A Renewable Resource

Although eternal growth is one of the central concepts of the United States and our economy, our land is finite. Like trust fund babies, we inherited a vast "savings deposit" of natural resources built up over millenia. This savings deposit only produces so much a year; if we withdraw too much of the resources without putting anything back in, we begin chipping away at the capital. If this continues, one day we'll find the planet has gone bankrupt.

In the past, farmers were careful with their land. They lived on it, and often it had been in their family for ages, so they were sure to sustain it for future generations by nourishing the soil and not depleting it. This sustainable agriculture largely ended with the modernization of farms and industry. Once we no longer lived on the farms or in the forests we lost the incentive to preserve them, and a once-in-a-billion-years spending spree on natural resources began which continues to this day. Our capital dwindles daily, and the need for sustainable agriculture grows.

Sustainable, ecological agriculture requires a revival of traditional multiple-crop cultivation using modern equipment and methods of harvesting and processing. Hemp, grown for fiber, is arguably the best choice for this purpose. Because hemp is easily biodegradable, its disposal presents no problems of waste management. The plant requires relatively little fertilizer in comparison with other fiber crops, and, having few natural predators, it

TABLE 1				
Hemp's Place in a Sustainable Crop Rotation				
1ST YEAR	2ND YEAR	3RD YEAR	4TH YEAR	5TH YEAR
Hemp Beets, Onions	Corn, Sugar	Wheat	Clover	Grass Potatoes
Corn	Peas, Beans	Hemp	Barley, Oats	Clover

needs little or no treatment with pesticides.

Almost every part of the hemp plant can be used by industry: the grain-like seed, strong fiber, and woody inner core known as the hurd. Hemp is a low-maintenance crop that can be grown in most climates, it does not deplete the soil of nutrients, and its deep root system can help to prevent erosion. It yields four times more fiber per acre than trees do, and it absorbs heavy-metal contaminants from soil, gradually purifying the earth. Since hemp plants grow 6 to 16 feet tall in 110 days, hemp is its own mulch; it shades out weeds and reduces the use of costly herbicides. Hemp yields three to eight tons of dry stalk per acre, depending on climate and variety. After hemp is harvested, the field is left virtually weed-free for the next crop. This last fact alone will save farmers thousands of dollars while improving water quality. Sustainable or organic growers can fertilize their hemp crops with biofertilizers such as compost, manures, and biosolids, and by planting nitrogen-fixing crops such as peas, beans, or clovers in rotation with hemp. Hemp tops and leaves, when returned to the field, add fertility to the soil.

Hemp benefits the environment and the rural economy while pro-

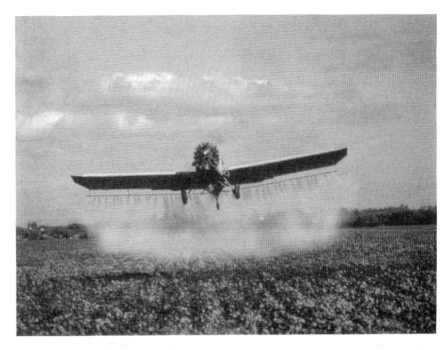

PESTICIDES AND HERBICIDES HAVE REACHED CRITICAL LEVELS OF CONTAMINATION IN MANY PARTS OF THE WORLD.

viding a sustainable alternative source of fiber for paper, textiles, and other purposes.

ROTTEN COTTON

Much of the groundwater tested in agricultural regions around the world has been contaminated by runoff from pesticides, herbicides, and fertilizers. Already 15,000 lakes in the United States are so contaminated that *nothing* can live in them. The potential health hazards from pesticides do not apply to wildlife alone. Tom Mount, in his book *World Medicine,* says

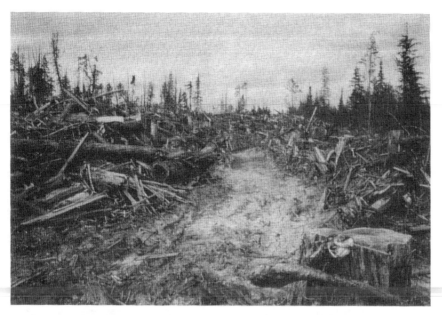

CLEARCUTTING, A PRACTICE THAT RUINS LAND AND WILDLIFE HABITAT FOR CENTURIES.

Farmers trusted the chemical companies' claims that the pesticides were harmless to humans, and perhaps they felt they had no choice but to use these chemicals given the realities of supporting their farms and families.

The pesticide king is cotton. Cotton is adapted to a wide range of uses, and it spins easily, but the environmental costs of cotton cultivation are incalculable. Cotton is grown on 3 percent of the earth's best arable land and uses a whopping 26 percent of the world's pesticides. It is a demanding crop that requires heavy irrigation and consumes more than 7 percent of the fertilizer used annually. It exhausts the soil, but is widely grown by developing countries desperate for a cash crop to repay international debts. Meanwhile, food crops are neglected, people go hungry, and the country's natural resources are destroyed. The large-scale monoculture of cotton around the Aral Sea in Russia has caused the sea to shrink as water is diverted from its tributary rivers, and the regional climate has changed accordingly. Many species of life have become extinct in that area, and the human population suffers from malnutrition and abnormally high levels of birth defects. Other areas in

that "farmers in the corn belt have the highest incidence of leukemia, prostate, and pancreatic cancer deaths," attributable to the "introduction of chlorinated hydrocarbon pesticides in 1945."

■■■

Much of the fiber for textiles currently comes from cotton. So what? Here's what:

- The *Wall Street Journal* has reported that many Asian cotton farmers use up to seven times the directed amount of pesticides for their crops.
- In the United States, about half the pesticides used today are sprayed on cotton plants.

- In 1993, two hundred and fifty thousand tons of pesticides were used to grow cotton worldwide. These pesticides wash into streams and rivers, destroying ecosystems and poisoning human water supplies.
- The June 1994 issue of *National Geographic* states that "in California alone some 6000 tons of pesticides and defoliants are used on cotton in a single year."

■■■

Africa, India, and the Americas suffer the same fate.[2]

With few insect enemies and little competition from weeds, hemp is a much better candidate than cotton to produce a high-quality, sustainable, and organically grown fiber.

TREE-FREE ALTERNATIVE

Deforestation is perhaps the most severe threat to the long-term health of the planet. 27,000 species of life go extinct every year, due largely to the 296 million acres (120 million hectares) of forest we have destroyed in the past twenty years. Already in North America we have lost 97 percent of the mature forest that greeted European settlers in the seventeenth century.[3] In addition to being primary habitat for the majority of life forms, forests are also vital to conserving the soil and to maintaining our air by removing carbon dioxide and returning oxygen. As our forests disappear, the delicate web of life frays closer to the breaking point.

Our demand for the products we now derive from wood—primarily paper, building supplies, and fuel—is increasing. America uses as much wood, by weight, as it uses metals, plastics, and cement combined. About 40 percent of the trees we destroy are used to make paper products such as wrapping and tissue paper. Some paper companies plant fast-growing eucalyptus trees after clearing the land and call that reforestation. The fallen eucalyptus leaves poison the soil so that nothing can grow there for many years after the trees are harvested. The replanting practices of logging companies are a poor substitute for natural forest because biodiversity is destroyed. Wildlife populations are much lower in tree plantations than in true forests. It is imperative that we move to a sustainable fiber to take wood's place.

THE HOUSE THAT HEMP BUILT

As any afficionado of antique furniture or old houses will tell you, they don't make wood the way they used to. This is simply a function of time: the three-hundred-year-old trees we took from the original forests were strong through competition; they could only grow incrementally as they competed for light and water, and their wood was dense because of that. Compared to old-growth trees, a twelve-year-old spruce in a tree farm is nothing but a glorified weed; it has freedom to grow

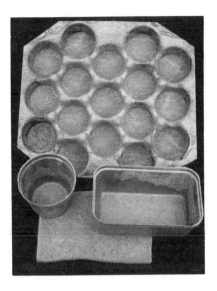

BOARDS AND CONTAINERS FROM HEMP HURDS. PHOTOGRAPH COURTESY OF INSTITUT FÜR ANGEWANDTE FORSCHUNG.

Hurds

The broken pieces of the woody core of hemp are called "hurds." They are a valuable commodity with many uses, including paper pulp, fiberboard, Isochanvre, planting substrate, nonwoven uses, biofilters, and animal bedding. Hurds are 50 percent more absorbent than wood chips, and they rapidly degrade in a compost heap. Hurds can be used for pulp paper, as feedstock for chemical products such as cellophane and rayon, and in many industrial materials.

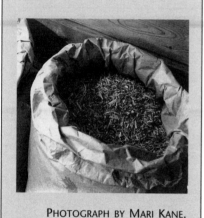

PHOTOGRAPH BY MARI KANE.

tall very quickly, and its wood is weak.

With timber becoming scarcer and prices skyrocketing, some in the industry now believe that wood will become a rare commodity that should be used only where it can be directly seen or touched, and an alternative product must be developed. To this end, the composite-board industry has become one of the fastest-growing segments of the wood-products industry. Composite boards are processed fiber held together with resins. When made from trees the boards are weak, since the individual fibers of trees are at best three-quarters of an inch long, so the boards can only replace lumber where strength is not required. Hemp fibers, on the other hand, run virtually the entire length of the plant—up to fifteen feet—and have expanded the horizons of the composite-board industry.

The major components of the hemp stalk are the long primary bast fiber, the shorter secondary fiber (tow), cellulose, hemicellulose, and lignin. Each of these has a particular place in the cycle of production. The outer fiber contains 60 to 78 percent cellulose, while the inner pulp, or hurd, is 36 to 41 percent cellulose and 31 to 37 percent hemicellulose. Fiber, primarily from the outer bast,

gives the composite hemp board strength and form. Cellulose, from the hurds, makes up the bulk. Lignin is an organic glue that can be extracted and used as a resin binder, replacing coventional binders that use formaldehyde.

Benefits of using hemp-based composites instead of trees include better resistance to fire, fungus, rodents, termites and other pests, in addition to the preservation of forests, stimulation of regional economies, and agricultural sustainability. Also, properly retted and stacked hemp can be stored for several years on end without significant deterioration, so the producer can take full advantage of changing markets.

To achieve a profitable economy of scale, a composite or fiberboard mill processes 1500 tons of raw material per day and operates 250 days a year. Its output is 375,000 tons of board per year. At six tons of dried stalk per acre that requires the seasonal output of 62,500 acres of hemp. (At $70 per ton, that pays the farmer $420 per acre.)

HEMP PAPER

Ever since hemp paper was invented by the Chinese about two thousand years ago, hemp has continued to be used for that purpose, and hemp textiles have been an essential source for rag paper. In a macabre instance, after World War II, the British paper manufacturer Robert Fletcher and Sons bought all the available Nazi concentration camp uniforms, which were made of hemp. Since then, the company has imported fiber from France because it is nearly impossible to obtain textiles that do not contain synthetic fibers, which ruin the paper-making machinery.

At present, only two dozen paper mills, mostly in China and India, with two in Europe, use hemp as a fiber source. The estimated volume of world production is about 120,000 tons of hemp-fiber pulp per year. By comparison, a typical single wood pulp mill produces at least 250,000 tons of pulp per year. Most hemp-fiber pulp is used for cigarette papers, filter papers, tea bags, art papers, and paper money.

Although the fiber content of cannabis is equal to or higher than most other competitive nonwood sources of paper pulp (such as sugarcane bagasse, retted flax, jute, bamboo, and cereal straws[4]), the qualities of hemp fiber are different from other pulp materials, and so require special beating and refining processing and equipment.

Announced in March 1994 in

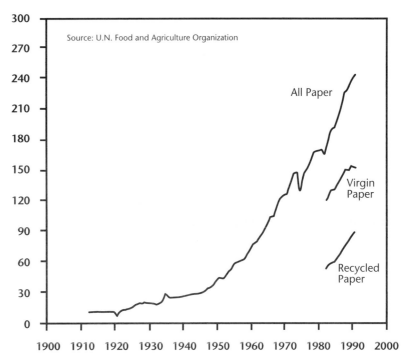

WORLD PAPER COMSUMPTION, 1913–91, AND RECYCLED PAPER CONSUMPTION, 1983–91. CHART COURTESY OF THE WORLDWATCH INSTITUTE.

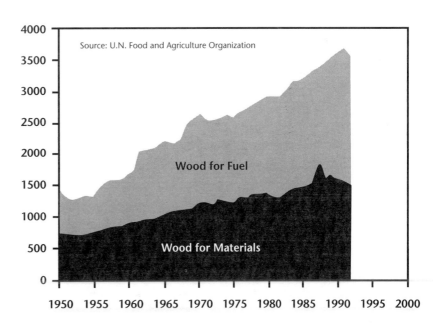

WORLD WOOD CONSUMPTION, 1950–91. CHART COURTESY OF THE WORLDWATCH INSTITUTE.

Cancer Valley, U.S.A.

Probably the greatest damage from paper mills is in their use of chlorine bleach to treat the lignin in wood. All fiber contains lignin, the natural glue that cements plant cell walls together. It is essential to remove the lignin content from cellulose to produce soft, white paper; if there is too much residual lignin, the fiber is brown and hard to handle. Delignification is done with chlorine, a compound that is extremely volatile and easily combines with hydrocarbons to produce organochlorides, a toxic family of substances such as DDT and chlordane. Organochlorides do not easily break down, and so move from our waters up through the food chain, accumulating in ever greater numbers in our own bodies. Recent evidence has shown that organochlorides likely cause irretrievable genetic damage to our immune and hormonal systems.[5] Dioxin, the chemical present in Agent Orange, is a by-product formed when pulp is treated with chlorine bleach. It is produced continuously by paper mills across the country. Communities near mills are reporting shockingly high levels of diseases, including cancer, nervous disorders, and liver damage. One area in Maine known to the locals as "Cancer Valley" has reported terrible rates of emphysema, asthma, lymphoma, lung cancer, leukemia, and aplastic anemia.[6]

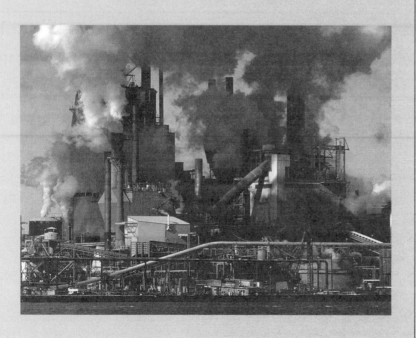

Frankfurt, Germany was the development of a closed-cycle ammonia-sulfite-alcohol (ASA) pulping process, which makes possible the production of hemp pulp without pollution. (Previously, as many as four chlorinations were necessary to delignify hemp cellulose.) The alcohol, water, and by-products from the process can be recovered for recycling or other applications. The selectivity and "soft" conditions of ASA-pulping enable bast fiber pulping to be separated into low-lignin long fibers and high-lignin short fibers. The ASA-pulping process makes possible the manufacture of hemp-hurd pulp equal in quality, 15 percent brighter, and much superior in yield to wood pulp. Another hemp-pulping technology developed in The Netherlands combines shear forces and small amounts of alkali and catalyst to remove more than 75 percent of the lignin from hemp fibers. (Conventional chemical methods remove only about 50 percent of the lignin.) Chemical-mechanical pulping makes possible the manufacture of hemp paper at a much lower cost than from wood.[7] Hydrogen peroxide is another possible substitute for chlorine in the bleaching process.

Hemp is not the only non-tree source of fiber, but it is the best.

While flax grows well in temperate climates (and has a cellulose content similar to that of hemp), the yield per acre is only about five hundred pounds, less than half that of hemp, and flax requires careful preparation of the soil. The Asian perennial ramie yields about 600 pounds per acre on well-drained land, but dry hot spells or cold snaps will kill the crop.

Jute produces a yield comparable with hemp, but it requires a warm humid climate, rich loam soil, and lots of rain during the growing season. Jute also exhausts the soil. Jute contains less cellulose than hemp, and is not well suited for papermaking because it does not bleach easily, and the bleached fibers disintegrate faster. Jute is cheap and plentiful and easy to spin, but it is the weakest and least durable of the major textile fibers.

After decades of research, the U.S. Department of Agriculture found the African hibiscus kenaf to be a superior fiber for papermaking. The yield of kenaf is low in cool climates, however; it can be cultivated in bulk only in countries where it is warm most of the year, and in the southern U.S. states of New Mexico, Texas, California, and Louisiana. More than any other competitive fiber plant, hemp grows well in many climates, including most of the

United States, and requires the least input of fertilizer, insecticides, herbicides, and attention. This makes it ideal for both the small family farm and the huge agro-business.[8]

Hemp As an Energy Resource

The application of industrial hemp with the greatest economic and social potential is also the use that has generated the most debate: its role in the multi-trillion-dollar energy industry.

While there is no question that hemp has been used as an energy source for centuries, current discussions center on its potential as an energy crop. To understand this situation, we must first consider the technical issues of using hemp as an energy resource, then take a closer look at its applications and economic scope.

Virtually any plant or organic matter (biomass) can be converted to fuel. Fuels derived from vegetable matter are known as biofuels. A University of Hawaii study reported in 1990 that biomass gasification could provide up to 90 percent of that state's energy needs.[9] Biofuels have several critical advantages over fossil fuels:[10]

- Plants contain almost no sulfur or a number of the other contaminants which are commonly found in petroleum and cause air pollution when burned as fuel. Sulfur is a major component in acid rain.
- Local agricultural crops can be converted into fuel. This makes energy more accessible, creates community jobs, and helps stimulate regional economic independence and autonomy.
- Plants use a chemical process known as photosynthesis to convert water and carbon dioxide (CO_2) into carbohydrates and oxygen. Since CO_2 is produced by burning fuel, biomass production essentially recycles this gas, the primary cause of global warming, back into a fuel source and thereby cleans the atmosphere.
- Harvesting plants does not require mining, strip-mining, or drilling and will not cause oil spills, so biomass production is better for the environment.
- Annual farm crops are *sustainable* fuel sources; they are renewed or replenished by a new crop each year, rather than being steadily drained or depleted, as are fossil fuels.

- It is possible to use agricultural, industrial, and municipal waste products as a raw material for fuel, thus reducing the solid waste that would otherwise present a disposal problem.

On the negative side of biofuels:

- Annual crops are harvested seasonally rather than year-round.
- Biomass is relatively bulky, which requires compaction and adds to storage and shipping costs.
- Considerable capital would need to be invested in the development of pyrolysis and incineration facilities.
- Plants require additional processing to be concentrated to the condition of fossil fuels.

All in all, the benefits of biofuel greatly outweigh its disadvantages. And once the feed stock has been converted into fuel, it fits right into the entire currently existing infrastructure of distribution and use: tankers, freight cars, pipelines, storage facilities, and so on. As time goes by, more and more of the energy industry is realizing that biomass is not just an option—it is the future.

Biomass can be processed into

a wide variety of liquid, solid, and gaseous fuels, which in turn can be used to produce electricity. One aspect that makes biomass particularly attractive is that the necessary technology already exists. The existing infrastructure can process, store, and transport biofuels with relatively little adaptation or modification.

Reliance on biofuels actually produces a significant economic gain from an ecological point of view, because the exploration, drilling, extraction, processing, and transportation of fossil fuels have all been eliminated and the end product is a cleaner-burning fuel. The main reason that fossil fuels seem to have a price advantage is that the cost of repairing the environmental damage is ignored. Why? Because the petrochemical energy producers know that it is cost-prohibitive to clean up after themselves, and their government allies simply let them off the hook. Similarly, the cost of military defense of oil fields is left out of the equation. At the same time, these companies get large tax breaks in the form of oil-depletion allowances on private holdings and subsidized access to publicly owned energy reserves. In short, the real costs are passed on to taxpayers without their knowledge or consent.

As the availability and quality of fossil fuels continues to deteriorate over the coming years, the price of energy will rise. As taxpayers learn more about the corporate welfare being doled out to multinational energy companies, they will demand that the government reduce or eliminate these handouts. The combined effect of these changes will be a more level field of competition, with greater economic and environmental incentives to switch over to biofuels. And that does not even take into consideration the health-care savings afforded by living in a cleaner environment.

Research into the potential for using enzymes to extract hydrogen from plant carbohydrates promises a very clean fuel (when hydrogen burns, its only by-product is H_2O—water!), but the process is expensive, and the technical infrastructure to use hydrogen effectively is not yet ready for mass production. Until that hurdle is cleared, the most practical approach seems to be to convert hemp and other biomass into conventional fuels.

In 1992, after studies at a pilot plant originally engineered for converting coal into gas, General Electric reported that biomass is a feasible fuel source. Researchers found that woody biomass had about half the heat value of an equal weight of coal and one-sixth that of natural gas, but they speculated that the real cost of electricity generated from biofuels would be lower due to savings in pollution-control systems. GE analyst Gene Kimura expressed concern that, due to concerns over global deforestation, biofuels would be politically viable only in conjunction with "some sort of forest management."

Why not leave the forests out of the equation and use an annual farm crop as a biofuel source? In that case, the best option is hemp. There are two major sources of biofuel to be derived from hemp: the seed oil and the stalk. We will consider each of these in turn.

HEMP SEED AS AN ENERGY SOURCE

Vegetable oils are superior to petroleum on several counts, and hemp seed produces one of nature's finest oils. It is also easily converted into diesel fuel. Since the oil is not intended for human consumption, rancid oil can be used. Chemical extraction processes can increase the overall oil yield to 40 percent of the seed volume. This fuel oil has traditionally been thinned and used in lamps, as well as for cooking and heating.

An average hemp seed harvest is twenty to thirty bushels per acre, each bushel weighing forty-four pounds. This leaves us with a range of 880 to 1320 pounds per acre, for an average of 1100 pounds per acre. (These figures are conservative. A study of feral hemp in Illinois arrived at a much higher seed yield estimate of four tons per acre, roughly eight times greater than the figures described here.[11])

If 35 percent of this weight is oil, the output is 385 pounds. Hemp-seed oil weighs about 8 pounds per gallon. This means a typical acre should yield about 48 gallons of seed oil (compared to 60 from safflower or sunflower), plus 715 pounds of seed cake, plus several tons of stalk. (An acre of seed hemp will produce less stalk weight and a lower quality fiber than will a fiber crop. Depending on the demand and the quality of the product, the seed cake and stalk can also be marketed as separate products or converted into fuel as described below.)

Hemp-seed oil has burning qualities and viscosity ratings similar to number-two heating oil. It is substantially thicker than processed liquid fuel and benefits from the addition of a small amount of methanol. This produces a premium oxygenated liquid fuel with a similar boiling range and viscosity to petroleum diesel fuel. Without this modification, hemp oil, like any vegetable oil, would cause excessive injector deposits. Once processed, however, this hybridized fuel source produces full engine power with reduced carbon monoxide and 75 percent less soot and particulates.

The critical issue here is not whether or not it is possible to produce energy this way, but whether other uses for the crop might be more profitable. For now at least the nutritional, lubricant, and fabrication value of the seed and its oil are more lucrative than the production of 50 gallons of fuel per acre. If, however, such fuel were to be used by farmers to run equipment, that self-sufficiency would reduce the overall cost of production and increase farm profitability.

HEMP STALK AS AN ENERGY SOURCE

On a yield-per-acre basis, including the hemp stalks as fuel is much more productive than limiting such development to the seed oil. Hemp roots and leafy matter enrich, aerate, and loosen the soil when left to preserve its vitality. Hemp's woody stalk can be removed and baled or bundled and

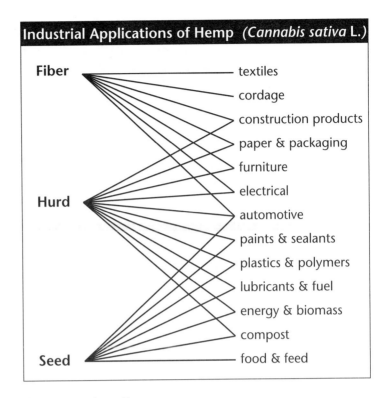

Industrial Applications of Hemp *(Cannabis sativa* L.)

Fiber — textiles, cordage, construction products, paper & packaging, furniture, electrical, automotive, paints & sealants, plastics & polymers, lubricants & fuel, energy & biomass, compost, food & feed

Hurd

Seed

COURTESY OF JOHN ROULAC.

burned directly for heat and to power boilers that generate electricity. The cellulose and hemicellulose in the core can be enzymatically or bacteriologically broken down into starches that can, in turn, be fermented into alcohol fuels or further digested into methanol, ethanol, or methane gas. Pioneered by the ancient Egyptians, pyrolysis can produce charcoal, noncondensable gases, acetic acid, acetone, methanol, and condensable organic liquids known as pyrolytic fuel oil. The technology can work with everything from fifty-five gallon drums to large processing plants.

With yields of five to ten tons of dried stalk per acre, energy farming could be a profitable enterprise.[12] Using the conservative, five-ton figure, we can extrapolate: Converting five tons of stalk will produce five hundred gallons of methanol per acre. At a wholesale rate of sixty cents per gallon, this comes to three hundred dollars gross per acre, slightly more than commonly grown crops like wheat or corn. On the other hand, buying those same five hundred gallons of fuel would cost the farmer about six hundred dollars. It therefore essentially doubles the value of the crop for the grower to use that fuel to offset the expenses of farming rather than to sell it at wholesale and then buy fuel on the retail market.

This seems to suggest cooperative development of small to mid-sized regional biomass conversion units, to which the growers bring raw or partially processed hemp for conversion in exchange for a steady supply of fuel. This could be done in conjunction with a decortication or other such facility so that the hemp crop is sorted, processed, and shipped out as value-added materials to the appropriate end user. That would afford farmers their highest profit potential, pro-vide manufacturers with ready-to-use materials, and lower transportation costs by eliminating initial bulk and later disposal costs of unwanted by-products.

One analysis predicts higher energy returns if producer gas is made through thermal gasification of the stalks.[13] Other options are hydrolization, diffraction, or various distillation processes.

Hemp As an Energy Crop

For hemp to provide all of the energy required by a country like the United States (or even a large percentage of it) would require millions of acres dedicated to hemp production. While some researchers consider the necessary scale of production unfeasible,[14] others contend that meeting U.S. demands for oil and gas would require intensive cultivation of only about 6 percent of the land area of the forty-eight contiguous states, or just over 116 million acres.[15] That land mass currently includes 422.2 million acres of cropland, 129 million acres of pasture, and 401.7 million acres of rangeland (this discounts all federal lands, urban development, and 393.9 million acres of rural forest). That means that just about 21 percent of these combined lands would have to be energy farms to supply the liquid fuel need for any given year.

This will be mitigated to some extent by the energy conversion of agricultural by-products (for example, manure, wheat straw, or whey from cheese) and urban solid waste (two tons of packaging waste produce about a ton of heating oil, but garbage also has additional contaminants to be removed). The Institute for Local Self-Reliance estimates 347.5 million tons of recoverable biomaterial waste is generated per year in the United States, the output equivalent of about 70 million acres of hemp.[16]

If about half of that could be recovered, it still leaves about 81 million acres of raw biomass to be grown each year, roughly 20 percent of available cropland. About 15 percent of cropland is now kept out of production, in part as fallow land to maintain soil viability and in part to keep the food supply down and keep prices up at a profitable level for the farmer. Hemp can be grown to rebuild soil or to eliminate weeds and soil pathogens, however, and since it would be used as fuel, it would not compete directly with other crops. Therefore, if two-thirds of that fallow land were used for energy farming, that would give America energy independence based on only 10 percent of current cropland being used for biofuels, or 42 million acres. This amount could also be divided between cropland and pasture so as to leave more land available for food production. This does not take into account use of undeveloped urban areas in vacant lots and industrial areas, which could also be used.

The bottom line is that it can be done, given the political will and economic investment, but it won't happen overnight. Growing hemp as an energy crop is a viable, long-term fuel alternative for the United States, which consumes about 60 percent of the planet's annual energy production. Hemp biofuels are even more practical for geographic areas that are less energy-intensive than North America.

From a global perspective, it has been argued that hemp is the superlative biomass crop (better than corn or trees, for instance) when sustainable ecological criteria are applied. Such criteria would require the following:

- Eliminate all chemical pesticides, herbicides, fertilizers, and other toxins.
- Limit cultivation to natural, organic processes.

- Include marginal land areas as well as prime farm land.
- Include rotational crops to maintain soil fertility and control pathogens.
- Factor in the water intake to crop output.
- Include all energy costs of cultivation and conversion.
- Eliminate all subsidies and environmental waivers.
- Include all costs of environmental repairs related to the production of the energy (such as air pollution, soil depletion, and chemical runoff).[17]

Energy As a Hemp By-product

The last time hemp was grown on a large scale in the United States, during World War II, on-site combustion of just 20 percent of waste materials was sufficient to power hemp-processing mills, with half of the energy produced being excess which was sold back to the power companies by the War Hemp Industries Corporation.[18] Theoretically, the remaining 80 percent could also be converted into energy and sold.

One deterrent to using hemp as a biofuel is that it is so valuable for its other uses. In the course of processing hemp into fiber or cellulosic pulp, however, a significant amount of waste is produced that has value as an energy-feed stock. If a manufacturer has an integrated system that utilizes all parts of the plant, this approach becomes a moot point because there is no waste.

Hemp's Practical Fuel Potential

All things considered, it appears that hemp does have good potential as a biofuel resource. In most cases, the value of the crop's fiber and seed will be greater than the value of energy it would produce. But waste produced at any point in the chain of production can be converted into fuel and utilized to offset the cost of buying energy.

By using hemp as a fuel source, energy companies may achieve significant savings in the installation and operation of pollution-control equipment. Companies already operating with other fuels could use hemp or hemp waste as a seasonal supplement to reduce overall operating costs and extend the available supply of other fuel sources.

Hemp biomass would be

especially important to Third World nations and people living in areas where other energy sources are scarce, or in communities that are so poor that the cost of fuel limits the ability to develop the local economy.

Neither hemp nor any other energy source is likely to become the only such resource used on a global level. The human family will continue to rely on a variety of fuel sources, including conservation and cogeneration to meet its energy needs. Hemp's ultimate role in the overall scheme of things will be determined by a wide range of regional and geopolitical factors, many of which are only now beginning to emerge. It would be shortsighted for society and industry to neglect the crop's energy potential.

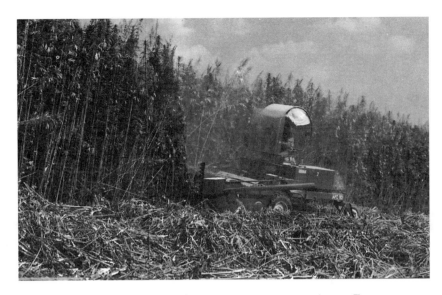

A MODERN HEMP FARM IN SPAIN. PHOTOGRAPH COURTESY OF LIVING TREE PAPER COMPANY.

Modern Hemp Husbandry

Early in the twentieth century, the U.S. Department of Agriculture encouraged domestic hemp production and in 1913 published its classic report "Hemp" by botanist Lyster H. Dewey.[19] Although the American hemp industry was virtually destroyed by the Marihuana Tax Act of 1937, farmers in China, India, Russia, Romania, Hungary, and France have continued to grow hemp for fiber. The U.N. Food and Agriculture Organization (FAO) reported that 260,000 hectares of hemp were cultivated in 1992. Cultivars have been developed that produce less than the legal limit of 0.3 percent THC, thus enabling the development of a fiber market without diversions for drug use.[20]

Meanwhile, the French hemp industry is developing under the aegis of a group of associations: Federation Nationale des Productions de Chanvre (FNPC), dedicated to agronomical research; and Comite Economique Agricole de la Production du Chanvre (CEAPC) and Cooperative Centrale des Producteurs de Semences de

Chanvre (CCPSC), both concerned with marketing hemp products. The three associations are directed by Jean-Paul Mathieu, and FNPC agronomist Olivier Beherec has bred several varieties of hemp suited for the European farming climate.

Britain lifted its ban on industrial hemp cultivation in February 1993 "to allow U.K. farmers to gain a share of the market currently occupied by our E.C. partners." A coalition of farmers calling itself Hemcore, Ltd. immediately and successfully grew six hundred hectares (fifteen hundred acres) of hemp in East Anglia. The hemp contained no more than 0.3 percent THC, and all the fields were required to be invisible from the road. The primary local use for the fiber is for livestock bedding, because it is extremely absorbent and composts easily. Any surplus has a ready market at paper mills and with foreign traders.

For the first time since 1937 Canadian farmers began to plant hemp for fiber in spring 1994. Alexander Sumach of the Hemp Futures Study Group congratulated the nation in the *Globe and Mail*:

> We are delighted to learn of the rebirth of the Canadian Hemp Industry. Farmer Joe Stroebel and engineer Geof Kime planted 20 hectares . . . with plump, innocent government approved hempseed from the finest European pedigrees. . . . It arrived not a minute too soon. The real treat is that Canadians actually beat Americans to this great prize. As the North American Free-Trade Agreement pretty well wiped out the last of a once-thriving Canadian textile industry, we should be glad that hemp is being planted. . . . There is nothing in NAFTA or the General Agreement on Tariffs and Trade about hemp. There is nothing to stop a great industry from taking off from Canadian soil. . . . The Americans will never get it together within the decade to grow hemp. Their laws will never admit that cannabis has any redeeming qualities.[21]

SOIL AND WATER

About twenty hours of labor per acre are required to produce a crop of hemp. This includes plowing, disking, harrowing, seeding, and rolling the acreage, then reaping, bundling, spreading, picking up, breaking, hackling, baling, and transporting the hemp.

Hemp loosens, mellows, and shades the soil, and the fallen foliage forms a mulch that preserves moisture and bacteria in the soil.

The root system penetrates deeply, and it decays quickly after the harvest. Up to two-thirds of the organic matter returns to the soil if hemp is field-retted (see below). Land is easier to plow after hemp than after small grains or corn. Hemp depletes some humus, but nonetheless is easier on the land than any other crops except legumes such as alfalfa and clover.

During World War II, the German government published *The Humorous Hemp Primer* to educate farmers about hemp and encourage its cultivation. The primer recommended moor land:

> He who grows hemp in the moor is carrying on true moor-culture since the options are quite limited: the moor farmer grows potatoes, cabbage, and some grains as well as corn. Little else can grow here. . . . Here the mighty hemp plant enters as saviour of the moor lands. It grows quick and large and helps cultivate the land. Most any crop is happy to alternate with hemp, since hemp's shady umbrella forces weeds to their knees. It keeps the moor ground dark, clean, and healthy. Also the moor's tendency to late rust doesn't bother hemp a bit. . . . Even virgin soil in the marsh can yield weak hemp production. However, when properly drained, hemp performance is quickly improved. In short, marsh values are increased by sowing hemp![22]

CULTIVATION

Hemp makes a perfect rotation crop with more traditional crops, enabling farmers to begin growing hemp without sacrificing their main source of income. The German *Humorous Hemp Primer* says that "hemp does well following almost any crop: It grows well after fruits, corn, vegetables, grasses and grains." Shady hemp is also an excellent preceding crop, according to the primer, because "its tall, wide, dense growth strangles weeds. After hemp, all grains grow well and without problems. Also, fruits which follow hemp bring larger crops, as do grasses, delicate and tender when they lie down in hemp's bed. In short, anything sown in hemp's fields will bring rich harvest and much money."

The USDA Farmers' Bulletin No. 1935 affirmed that "old pastures plowed up [in the fall] are well suited for hemp culture. Fields previously cropped to soybeans, alfalfa, and clover are excellent for hemp. A good rotation is to follow corn with hemp, and in Kentucky a fall cereal may follow the hemp."

Narrow crop rotation increases

> ■ ■ ■
> Bee keepers use hemp as a pollen insulator; no other plant is so efficient as a hedge against unwanted pollination.
> ■ ■ ■

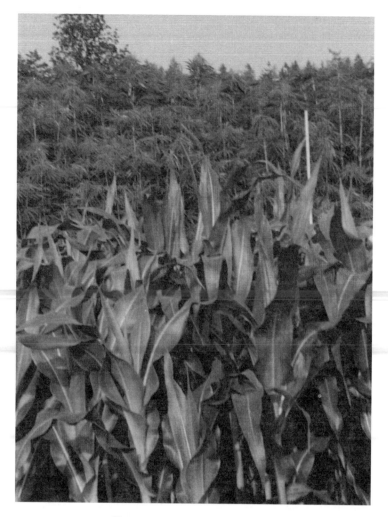

HEMP AND CORN: A PERFECT ROTATION. PHOTOGRAPH COURTESY OF SWIHTCO.

presses weeds, and is nearly free of diseases and pests. In ordinary schemes of crop rotation, hemp can occupy the same place as oats or beans. Hemp seems to be an excellent green manure for wheat.

As a companion plant, cannabis protects against the white cabbage butterfly and guards potatoes from late blight by *Phytophtora infestans.* Beans grown together with hemp will not become infested with brown spot. Hemp is effective against infestation of asters by *Fusarium,* protects sugar beets from turnip fleas, and guards peas from pea aphids *(Acyrthosiphon pisum).* Weevils are not likely to become established in granaries where hemp has been dried.

With the dangers of cigarette smoking becoming more and more apparent, the tobacco industry is in the beginning of what promises to be a steep decline, and there is a strong interest among tobacco farmers in the cultivation of hemp. There are some obstacles facing potential hemp farmers; it's an unfamiliar crop, and most hemp markets are still in their infancy. The majority of hemp grown today still relies on plentiful labor rather than mechanized harvesting equipment, so industrial countries will need to invest in the design of new farm

the incidence of diseases and soil pathogens, resulting in lower yields and the need for increased use of soil fumigants and other biocides. The introduction of hemp as a new crop into the cycle of rotations can help solve such problems. This high-yield crop improves soil structure, sup-

machinery before large-scale plantings will be cost-efficient.[23] But the main tobacco belt across the southestern U.S. is so ideal a climate for hemp that the tobacco farmer hesitant to make a change would do well to heed the words of hemp farmer John Bordley, recorded for posterity in 1799:

> My hemp never suffered materially from drought but once, and that of a sowing in May. . . . If the ground be good and well prepared, no crop is more certain than Hemp sowed in time and when the soil is moist. But, how uncertain is the tobacco crop! Failure of plants from frost, drought, or fly; want of seasonable weather for planting; web-worm, horn-worm; buttening low, for want of rain; curling or frenching, from too much rain; house-burning or funking whilst curing; frost before housed; heating in bulk or in the hogshead; inspection, culling, &c. Cultivating tobacco cleans, but exposes the soil to exhalation and washing away. It is only about a month that it shelters the ground: but Hemp shades it from May 'till about the first of August. . . .
>   A planter gaining 20 hogsheads of tobacco from 20 acres of ground, value 800 dollars, might expect 12,000 or 16,000 lbs. of Hemp from the same ground, value 1,000 or 1,200 dollars. But, if the income from Hemp should be a fourth less than from the tobacco crop, yet I would, on several accounts, prefer the hemp culture.

Hemp cultivation presents only a few common problems. When hemp is cultivated for seed, Canada thistles may appear in dense stands and must be spudded out while the hemp is only a few inches high—but Canada thistle and quack grass can be completely eradicated by one crop of hemp. Seedling hemp may be attacked by cutworms and white grubs, especially after a spring plowing. Wild morning glory and bindweed vines will climb up hemp stalks. Hemp is sorely bothered by parasitic broomrape *(Orobanche ramosa),* a very short plant with yellowish leaves and dull purple flowers. Broomrape roots are parasitic on the roots of hemp, killing plants before they mature. Broomrape can be controlled by diligent crop rotation and clean seeds.

RETTING

Previous to this century the greatest obstacle to large-scale hemp farming was the labor involved in separating the highly fibrous bast (outer bark) from the hurds. This

Electro-Culture

The application of electricity, magnetism, monochrome light, and sound can greatly stimulate the growth of plants. This little-known technology, called electro-culture, can accelerate growth rates, increase yields, improve crop quality, protect plants from diseases, insects, and frost, and reduce the requirements for fertilizer and pesticides. Two Soviet researchers reported that "under the influence of the electric current, the numerical proportions between hemp plants of different sexes was changed by comparison with the control to give an increased number of female plants by 20–25 percent, in connection with a reduction in the intensity of the oxidative processes in the plant tissues." Reports that the characteristics acquired by the plants in electrically treated soil are transmitted by inheritance to the third generation are particularly interesting.[24]

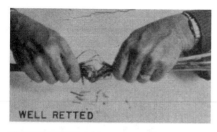

WELL RETTED

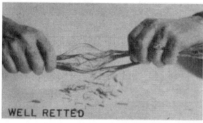

WELL RETTED

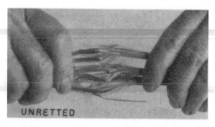

UNRETTED

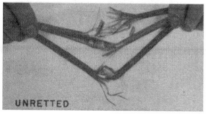

UNRETTED

UNTIL THIS CENTURY, RETTING WAS THE ONLY MEANS FOR SEPARATING THE OUTER FIBER OF HEMP FROM THE INNER PULP. PHOTOGRAPHS FROM USDA FARMERS' BULLETIN NO. 1935.

was accomplished by retting. Retting is the partial rotting of hemp stalks to enable the bast fibers to separate from the hurds. Dew-retting (or field-retting) is accomplished by spreading stalks on the ground to be exposed to rain and dew. In some parts of China and Japan, hemp fiber is prepared by soaking the stalks for one or two days, then steaming the stalks for three hours, then peeling off the fiber and scraping it to remove the outer skin. The resulting product is a stiff ribbon that is not well suited for spinning.

When retting is complete, the stalks are dried and sorted by grades, then crushed in a manual hemp-break, a wooden press of intersecting boards that break the stalks so the hurds can be removed.

An acre of hemp yields an average of fifteen thousand pounds of green stalks. After drying and curing in shocks, the stalks weigh about five tons. After retting and drying, the stalks weigh about three tons, and they yield about 750 pounds of long, rough fiber. The yield of hurds is about 2.5 tons per acre.

Hemp Technology

THE SCHLICHTEN DECORTICATOR

Hundreds of hemp-processing machines have been patented since Thomas Jefferson recorded his invention of an improved hemp-break (see chapter 5), but only the decorticator perfected by George W. Schlichten worked efficiently enough to meet the needs of the industry. The Schlichten decorticator could strip the fiber from nearly any plant, leaving the pulp (or hurds) behind. The machine promised to revolutionize the hemp industry by completely eliminating the need for retting.

As described in Schlicten's U.S. Patent #1,308,376 (1 July 1915), "the fiber produced is at once ready and suitable for carding or combing without any further treatment such as degumming or retting, and leaving the fiber soft, pliant, adhesive and in its unimpaired natural strength and color." In 1916, after eighteen years of development and a four-hundred-thousand-dollar investment, Schlichten tested the market for the "sliver" of hemp fiber his machine produced. He sold his entire first batch to a spinning mill owned by John D. Rockefeller and was paid a record premium of one hundred dollars a ton. Afterward the mill offered to buy the exclusive rights to the invention, and at a higher price than Schlichten had wanted, but he declined the offer.

Field-dried stalks are introduced to the Schlichten decorticator on a corrugated feed table or through revolving disks that serve to keep the stalks separated and straight. The stalks pass through fluted crushing and denting rollers, then through splitting and spreading rollers. The stalks then pass between a series of primary and secondary breaker rollers. Next, a high-speed rotating coarse comber begins to clean the fiber and degums it by separating the nonfibrous products, along with the short "tow" fibers. Corrugated softening rolls then soften the fiber and hold it in position for another series of combing and softening rollers. Finally, an endless slatted carrier eliminates any remaining small waste particles and delivers the fiber in an endless, folded "sliver" that is ready to be hanked and baled, and is prepared for any application.[25]

Schlicten's decorticator came to the attention of industrialist Henry H. Timken (inventor of the roller bearing), who was impressed by its possibilities. Timken arranged to meet Schlichten in February

THE SCHLICTEN DECORTICATOR.

1917 to secure the rights to the machine, and offered him the use of one hundred acres of his ranchland in Imperial Valley, California, to grow a crop of hemp to test on the decorticator. Timken also tried to interest newspaper magnate

■ ■ ■

In 1916, the United States Department of Agriculture published Bulletin No. 404: "Hemp Hurds As Paper-Making Material," written by Lyster H. Dewey and Jason L. Merrill and printed on hemp paper. George Schlichten, who had recently invented a hemp decorticator, provided Merrill, a paper-plant chemist, with hemp hurds. Merrill conducted hundreds of experiments to develop the prototype process for production of hemp-hurd paper. Eventually he produced a product that got a nod of approval from experienced paper makers.

Even in 1916, Dewey and Merrill's report sounded a warning that has become familiar in the late twentieth century: "There appears to be little doubt that under the present system of forest use and consumption the present supply can not withstand the demands placed upon it. By the time improved methods of forestry have established an equilibrium between production and consumption, the price of wood pulp may be such that a knowledge of other available raw materials may be imperative." The report determined that every tract of 10,000 acres that was devoted to hemp raising would, on a year-by-year basis, be equivalent to a sustained pulp-producing capacity of 40,500 acres of average pulp-wood lands.

■ ■ ■

Edward W. Scripps and his associate Milton McRae in the idea of making newsprint from hemp hurds.

In 1914 the circulation of daily newspapers had increased to more than 28 million copies and supplying newsprint was an increasing concern. Schlicten had investigated many kinds of plants for possible use in making paper, including corn and cotton. He found that hemp hurds could be made into a paper of higher grade than ordinary news stock.

Letters and interviews in the Scripps Collection at Ohio University Archives in Athens record the negotiations over the enormous potential of the decorticator. In one interview Schlichten, speaking on hemp-hurds paper stock, said, "The time will come when wood cannot be used for paper any more. It will be too expensive or forbidden. We have got to look for something that can be produced annually. . . . It takes twelve years before you have an acre grown into spruce; in twelve months I have a harvest of fifty tons produced. . . . It is actually a crime to chop down trees to get a small percentage of paper."

Schlichten's 1917 bumper crop of 14- to 16-foot-tall hemp attracted national attention and coverage from the major newsreel companies. Unfortunately for America and the world at large, the economic impact of World War I, high taxes, and other considerations deterred Scripps, McRae, and Timken from financing the Schlichten decorticator. Despite this setback, Schlichten persevered with his marvelous machine and it was rediscovered by the industry in 1937 and given the public attention it deserved, albeit too late. The Marihuana Tax Act of 1937 effectively aborted the renaissance of the hemp industry. Schlichten died a ruined man, and America's future was tragically altered.

RECENT DEVELOPMENTS

In the 1990s several developments and innovations in hemp-fiber processing have emerged that make it all the more eco-friendly. The new technologies produce high yields of standard-quality fiber at competitive prices for industrial purposes. The high-tensile strength of hemp fiber makes it suitable as a low-density reinforcing material in applications such as fiberglass. The absorptive properties, temperature stability, and biodegradability can be modified by pretreatments such as drying, carbonizing, impregnation, and mineralization.

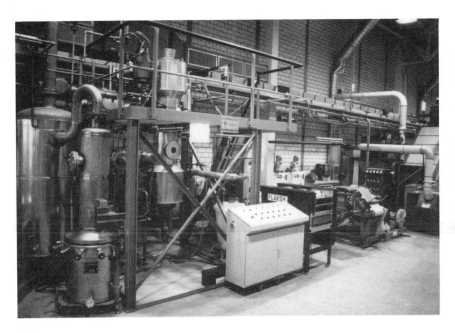

THE STEAM-EXPLOSION PROCESS: THE MARRIAGE OF HIGH-TECH SCIENCE AND AN ANCIENT PLANT. PHOTOGRAPH COURTESY OF INSTITUT FÜR ANGEWANDTE FORSCHUNG.

For example, the German company Ecco Gleittechnik has developed Iso-Hanf, a hemp fleece impregnated with sodium silicate and borate for fire resistance. The use of Iso-Hanf to reinforce concrete increases its flexibility by 30 percent. The drying characteristics and strength of mortar also are improved by Iso-Hanf. Its use in paint increases viscosity and resistance to detergents, and reduces the number of microfissures.[26]

C&S Specialty Builders Supply and Xylem Inc. have developed a prototype "Xylanizer," using steam explosion to reduce the hemp plant to cellulose, hemicellulose, and lignin, eliminating the need for retting or decortication.

These and other modern applications for hemp have given us the potential to change our vision of the future. A world now beckons around the corner where soil is being purified, forests are slowly marching back, the air is cleaner, and farmers are going back to their farms. If this sounds impossible, that only shows how far we have fallen, how jaded we've become. A clean environment *and* healthy jobs is no pipe dream, it is the base on which our collective sanity rests. We had it for millenia, now we've lost it. Hemp is the first and biggest step to getting it back.

2

HEMP
AND
HEALTH

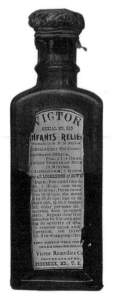

When we hear pleas to preserve nature—the forest, the water—they don't always hit home. Sure, protecting the environment sounds great, but it's not a part of *our* lives. What's a clearcut in Maine or a hole in the ozone over Antarctica got to do with us?

But this division between nature and us is a product of our minds, and it is no coincidence that every damage we inflict upon the heavenly body we inhabit is reflected within ourselves. Clearcuts tear into our forests, and strange new cancers ravage our bodies. Species go extinct, and human sperm counts plummet. Dioxins wash down our waterways and into our bloodstreams. The pesticides on our cotton fields may wash away—but where is away?

We eat, drink, and breathe nature every minute of every day. It comes as no shock, then, to learn that the same plant proving to be a key to healing and sustaining our world has been sustaining our bodies for centuries. Hemp has been known as a valuable healing plant in every region where it will grow. It has been used to treat digestive disorders, neuralgia, insomnia, depression, migraines, and inflammation. Women have used it to facilitate childbirth, stimulate lactation, and relieve menstrual cramping.

The first documented use of hemp as medicine appears about 2300 B.C.E.,

EARLY AMERICAN CHILDREN'S MEDICINE CONTAINING CANNABIS. PHOTOGRAPH BY ANDRE GROSSMAN.

when the legendary Chinese emperor Shen Nung prescribed *chu-ma* (female hemp) for the treatment of constipation, gout, beri-beri, malaria, rheumatism, and menstrual problems. Shen Nung classified *chu-ma* as one of the Superior Elixirs of Immortality.

Chinese herbalists recommend *huo ma ren* ("fire hemp seeds") in doses from 9 to 15 grams, up to 45 grams, to nourish the yin (the feminine) in cases of constipation in the elderly, "blood deficiency," and recuperation from febrile diseases. In Chinese medicine hemp seed falls under the categories "sweet," "neutral," and "clears heat," operating through the channels of the stomach, large intestine, and spleen. It promotes the healing of sores and ulcerations when applied topically or ingested. Excessive or prolonged use may result in "vaginal discharge" or spermatorrhea. In China, the oil of hemp in a mixture of herbal extracts is widely sold for use as a laxative.[1]

Both the ancient Ayurvedic system of Indian medicine and the Arabic Unani Tibbi system make extensive use of hemp for healing. Usually, it is mixed with other vegetable, mineral, and animal substances that neutralize the narcotic effects and enhance the therapeutic powers. The tenth

---

The *Pen T'sao Kang Mu* (or *Ben Gao Gang Mu*) was written during the Ming dynasty by the physician Li Shi-Chen (1573–1620 C.E.). It is still the most extensive treatment of Chinese materia medica available. A section relating to postpartum constipation and chill reads as follows:

> After giving birth to a child, there is often instances of copious and constant Sweating, and a direct influence upon the Large Intestine, so that there is also developed a propensity toward Constipation. The patient is the type who hates to use medicines of any kind or reacts adversely, or is having complications from other medication and treatment to the point that they strenuously resist efforts to settle themselves down.

> The simple cure for this is that the use of a gruel made up from [Hemp Seed] will produce a very strong Calming effect on the patient. Also it should be stated that this is not only a good formula to take in the case of conditions arising from the complications of giving birth.

Translation by Norman Goundry

---

century treatise *Anandakanda* describes fifty preparations of bhang for cures, rejuvenation, and as an aphrodisiac.

Ayurvedic physicians of India use bhang to treat dozens of diseases and medical problems including diarrhea, epilepsy, delirium and insanity, colic, rheumatism, gastritis, anorexia, consumption, fistula, nausea, fever, jaundice, bronchitis, leprosy, spleen disorders, diabetes, cold, anemia, menstrual pain, tuberculosis, elephantiasis, asthma, gout, constipation, and malaria. Other preparations of hemp are used to induce sleep, as a diuretic, and against hydrophobia (rabies), blood in the urine, hemorrhoids,

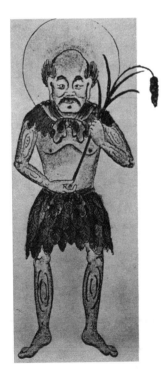

CHINESE EMPEROR SHEN NUNG, AUTHOR OF THE OLDEST KNOWN PHARMACOPOEIA.

hay fever, asthma, and skin diseases.[2]

Hemp was a popular folk remedy in medieval Europe, and it received honorable mention as a healing plant in herbals such as those by William Turner, Mattioli, and Dioscobas Taberaemontanus. Nicholas Culpepper (1616–1654) advised in his herbal that "an emulsion or decoction of the seed . . . eases the colic and always the troublesome humours in the bowels and stays bleeding at the mouth, nose, and other places."

In the middle of the nineteenth century, Dr. William O'Shaughnessy, a professor of chemistry at the Medical College of Calcutta, helped introduce cannabis, which he encountered as "bhang," to European medicine. As he described it,

> The Majoon or hemp confection, is a compound of sugar, butter, flour, milk, and *siddhi,* or bhang. . . . Almost invariably the inebriation is of the most cheerful kind, causing the person to sing and dance, to eat food with great relish, and to seek aphrodisiac enjoyments. In persons of a quarrelsome nature it occasions, as might be expected, an exasperation of their natural tendency. The intoxication lasts about three hours, when sleep supervenes. No nausea or sickness of the stomach succeeds, nor are the bowels at all affected; next day there is slight giddiness and vascularity of the eyes, but no other symptoms worth recording.

O'Shaughnessy gave a detailed account of the use of hemp resin (two grains every hour) to alleviate the suffering of a man dying of hydrophobia: "[I]t seems evident that at least one advantage was gained from the use of the remedy—the awful malady was stripped of its horrors; if not less fatal than before, it was reduced to less than the scale of suffering which precedes death from most ordinary diseases."[3]

Hemp soon became an official member of the pharmaceutical repertoire in Europe and America. The pharmaceutical preparation called Squire's Extract was commonly used as a specific to alleviate the symptoms of tetanus, typhus, and hydrophobia.

Pharmacists found cannabis useful, with varying degrees of success, for all of the maladies the Indians and Chinese had long been treating with hemp. They also found it effective in the treatment of alcoholism, dysentery, uterine hemorrhage, migraine, palsy, anthrax, blood poisoning, incontinence, leprosy, snakebite, tonsilitis, parasites, and a legion of other medical problems.[4]

Reports of "cannabis poisoning" occasionally surfaced, but as one physician noted in a 1912 essay on hashish, "Not one authenticated case is on record in which [an overdose of] cannabis or any of its preparations . . . [has] produced death in man or the lower animals." That record holds true to date.[5] In fact, one of the most remarkable qualities of cannabis is its safety as a medicine. With a lethal-to-effective-dose ratio of 40,000 to 1, cannabis is far safer than aspirin and most other legal medicines, which commonly have a lethal dose only ten times greater than their effective one.[6]

In the late nineteenth century, cannabis was included in dozens of remedies available by prescription or over the counter. Among them were the stomachic Chlorodyne, and Corn Collodium, manufactured by Squibb Company. Parke-Davis made Casadein, Utroval, and Veterinary Colic Medicine, and Eli Lilly produced Dr. Brown's Sedative Tablets, Syrup Tolu Compound, Syrup Lobelia, Neurosine, and One Day Cough Cure. The company of Grimault and Sons marketed cannabis cigarettes as a remedy for asthma. The use of a now illegal product by what are some of the largest pharmaceutical companies in the world is no more surprising than the cocaine used in Coca-Cola in the early part of the century, and it emphasizes the arbitrary nature of "controlled substances." Far from being the enemies of civilization the Drug Enforcement Agency likes to depict, these are natural substances subject to the whims of government: mainstay in the home medicine cabinet today, sinister corruptor of children tomorrow.

The eventual decline in use of cannabis by these firms was not due to any crisis of conscience. Rather, they were unable to stabilize or standardize any form of preparation of cannabis extracts, thus there was no profit in it. Undoubtedly today the wide availability and inexpensiveness of cannabis has kept these firms from showing any new interest in it and using their powerful influence with the Food and Drug Administration.

With the institution of its prohibition, cannabis was removed from the British pharmacopoeia in 1932. It was censored from the U.S. pharmacopoeia in 1942 and the *Merck Index* deleted its listing for cannabis in 1950. The Indian pharmacopoeia continued to list cannabis until 1966. Yet, despite all the suppression, propaganda, and denials by the United States

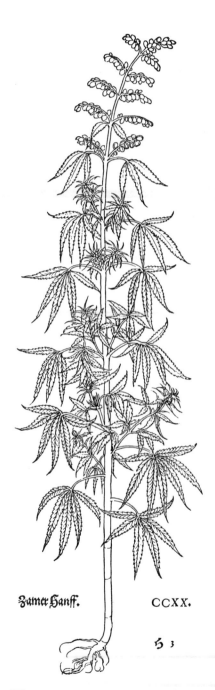

WOODCUT OF HEMP AS ILLUSTRATED IN THE HERBAL *KREUTERBUCH* OF LEONARD FUCHS, 1543.

Cannabis and Night Vision

M. E. West of the Department of Pharmacology at the University of the West Indies confirmed the Jamaican folk belief that a rum-extract of cannabis improves night vision when he accompanied the crew of a fishing boat on a dark night: "At daybreak it was impossible to believe that anyone could navigate a boat without compass and without light in such treacherous surroundings. I was then convinced that the man who had taken the rum extract of cannabis had far better night vision than I had, and that a subjective effect was not responsible. Note that the fisherman allowed about half an hour to an hour to elapse before setting out to sea after taking the extract. And I was told that the effect on their vision was the same whether they smoked the cannabis or took the extract."

Dr. West and Dr. Albert Lockhart, an opthalmologist, eventually prepared a nonpsychoactive substance, called Canasol, which showed a marked effect on intraocular pressure (IOP) and "significant improvement in night vision." West speculated that adrenoreceptors are involved, possibly located in the ciliary epithelium.[7]

and other governments, people have continued to rediscover the medical effects of smoking cannabis, and hundreds of scientific articles have been published reporting its health benefits.

Therapeutic Uses

Medical research as well as anecdotal evidence supporting the therapeutic applications of the major cannabinoids—tetrahydrocannabinol (THC), cannabinol (CBN), and cannabidiol (CBD)—is voluminous.

For glaucoma. Several million people worldwide are afflicted with glaucoma, an incurable disease of the eyes in which the unchecked rise of intraocular pressure (IOP) causes irreparable damage of the retina and optic nerve, resulting in blindness. Glaucoma is somewhat controllable with medications, all of which are attended by dangerous side-effects—with the exception of cannabis.[8] In one important report from 1971, researchers R. S. Hepler and I. M. Frank chanced to notice that the smoking of cannabis reduced IOP by about 25 percent after thirty minutes. In addition, there was a 50 percent reduction in tear flow and ocular pulse pressure, with no development of tolerance. The effect occurs with THC and cannabis extracts administered orally, intravenously, or by topical application.[9]

As an anti-emetic. In the 1970s, patients undergoing chemotherapy for Hodgkin's disease and other cancers discovered that if they smoked cannabis before receiving chemotherapy, they suffered less nausea and vomiting. The side-effects of the cannabis—being "high," dysphoric, or sedated, for instance—seem to be tolerated better by young persons than older patients. A study reported in the *New England Journal of Medicine* indicated that nausea and vomiting was controlled by THC in 81 percent of patients.[10]

Chemotherapy patients who use hemp as medicine generally prefer to smoke cannabis rather than ingest synthetic THC (Marinol) because they usually vomit before the pill can take effect (up to three hours later). Smoking allows the patient to titrate the dose puff by puff, and the medicine takes effect within a few minutes. Synthetic THC also loses its effectiveness after only a few treatments and is expensive. One effective method of ingesting cannabis is to prepare an extract with clarified butter, administering it in suppository capsules with pinholes poked in them.

A 1990 Harvard University survey of members of the American Society of Clinical Oncology revealed that 44 percent of the 1035 respondents acknowledged they had recommended the illegal use of cannabis to at least one patient undergoing chemotherapy for cancer. Nearly half the respondents agreed that they "would prescribe cannabis in smoked form to some of their patients if it were legal."[11]

For Breathing Difficulty. For at least three thousand years cannabis has provided relief for asthmatics, and it was widely used for

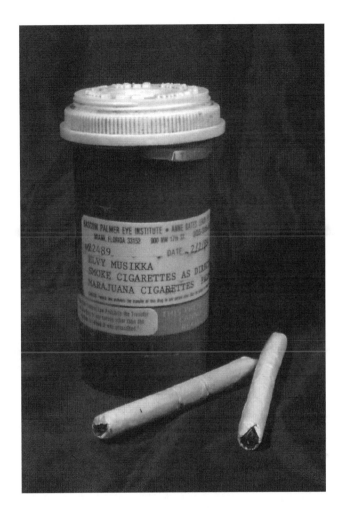

A RARE SIGHT: LEGALLY PRESCRIBED CANNABIS. PHOTOGRAPH BY ANDRE GROSSMAN.

that purpose especially in the nineteenth century. The inhalation of cannabis smoke causes bronchial dilation lasting up to one hour. The bronchodilator effect of orally ingested THC lasts up to six hours, but is not so powerful as smoking cannabis. THC aerosols are not as effective as smoking cannabis because aerosolized THC has an irritating effect on the air passages.[13]

THC in a microaerosol has proved to be up to 60 percent effective as a bronchodilator, with minimal mental effects and no parasympathetic effects.[14] Other research demonstrates that THC defends against the encroachment of emphysema[15] and suppresses coughing.[16] Cannabis has been used successfully in the treatment of whooping cough.[17]

As an anticonvulsant. The power of cannabis to control spasticity and convulsions has been known to folk medicine for millennia. The first European report of this effect was published by Dr. William O'Shaughnessy, who stated that "The [medical] profession has gained an anti-convulsive remedy of the greatest value."[18]

Many thousands of victims of all forms of convulsions, spasticity, and epilepsy, of forms of paralysis including paraplegia, quadriplegia, muscular dystrophy (MD), and multiple sclerosis (MS), and of chorea and associated neuralgias praise cannabis for its unique relaxant power. Anecdotal reports of its effectiveness prompted clinical studies that showed that Cannabidiol (CBD) can help many patients to remain nearly free of convulsions without any toxicity, behavioral

impairment, or tolerance. One researcher found a "limited effect" of smoking cannabis to alleviate the spasticity of MS[19] and others have found THC also to be useful in the treatment of muscular dystrophy.[20]

To inhibit tumors. THC and CBN have been found to inhibit Lewis Lung Tumor.[21] THC and CBN inhibited primary tumor growth from 25 percent to 82 percent and increased the life expectancy of cancerous mice to the same extent. The anti-tumor property of THC and CBN is very selective, as it reduces tumor cells without damaging normal cells.[22]

As an antibiotic. Cannabinoid acids effectively inhibit and kill gram-positive bacteria such as staphylococci and streptococci. An alcoholic extract of cannabis has been recommended as a topical application and for use in the treatment of penicillin-resistant organisms. One group of researchers reported a case in which a pathologist injured his thumb during a dissection. It became severely infected and was absolutely resistant to other antibiotics. Amputation was imminently necessary, but the infection was defeated at the last minute by an application of cannabis extract.[23] Herpes labialis (recurrent viral inflammation of the oral mucous membranes), otitis media (inflammation of the middle ear), and second-degree burns have been treated successfully in the same way. The preparations of cannabis can be applied to the skin or mucous membranes as a salve, poultice, or spray.[24]

As an antiarthritic. Pliny the Elder recommended cannabis in the treatment of arthritis. In his *Treatise on Hemp,* M. Marcandier also mentioned that "the root of it boiled in water, and applied in the form of a cataplasm, softens and restores the joints or fingers or toes that are dried or shrunk. It is very good against the gout, and other humours that fall upon the nervous, muscular, or tendinous parts." Jamaicans use ganja for the same purpose.

The *Times of London* reported in 1994 that "the demand for cannabis among British pensioners has stunned doctors, police and suppliers . . . The old people use the drug to ease the pain of such ailments as arthritis and rheumatism. Many are running afoul of the law for the first time in their lives as they try to obtain supplies."[25]

As an antidepressant. As early as 1843, Jacques-Joseph Moreau de Tours extolled the value of hashish in the treatment of melancholy. In his *Hashish and Mental Illness,* Moreau wrote: "One of the effects of hashish that struck me most

forcibly and which generally gets the most attention is that manic excitement always accompanied by a feeling of gaiety and joy inconceivable to those who have not experienced it. . . . It is really happiness that is produced."[26]

In 1944 Dr. George Stockings reported on the synthetic cannabinoid Synhexyl as "a new euphoriant for depressive mental states," particularly in the treatment of neurotic depression, the most common psychiatric condition encountered in clinical practice. Stockings concluded, "Its use is not contraindicated by the presence of coexisting organic disease, and it is suitable for out-patient practice. Its use does not interfere with other therapeutic measures, such as occupational therapy or psychotherapy. It is free from risks and disadvantages of the more drastic forms of treatment."[27]

The results of more recent clinical studies regarding THC and depression have been inconsistent, but it is clear that many depressed out-patients who do not respond well to standard treatments find respite in cannabis.[28]

To control inflammation. The soothing effect of cannabis on inflammatory disorders has been known for centuries. In modern times cannabis has received recognition from physicians after some patients reported that smoking cannabis gave them relief from conditions such as pruritus and atopic dermatitis, an allergic reaction distinguished by severe itching and patches of inflamed skin. Conventional treatments with steroids and antihistamines have only a limited effect in controlling the problem, which can become life-threatening and disfiguring when it is complicated by infection.

Researchers have shown that THC has an antihistamine effect,[29] and also that an alcohol extract of cannabis augments aspirin's ability to reduce fever.[30] The *European Journal of Pharmacology* published results of a study indicating that oral administration of THC is twenty times more powerful than aspirin and twice as potent as hydrocortisone in its power to inhibit edema.[31] CBD was found to produce over 90 percent inhibition of erythema at a dose of only one hundred micrograms (THC produced only 10 percent inhibition).[32] A 1990 U.S. patent describes a simple aqueous mixture of calcium hydroxide and hempseed oil, used as a treatment for burns, bedsores, and other skin afflictions.[33]

As an analgesic. For thousands of years, cannabis preparations have been used to relieve pain. Several modern studies have shown analgesic effects of cannabis and its derivatives and analogues in animals, but the human model gives conflicting results. An alcohol extract of cannabis will enhance the effects of other analgesics.[34–36]

At a low dose, THC increases the analgesic effect of morphine by 500 percent. At double the dose of THC, morphine's effect is ten times greater. According to Sandra Welch, "One major advantage to a cannabis-morphine combination would be to reduce both the morphine component and a major morphine side effect, depression of the respiratory system. It has already been confirmed that cannabis has no effect on the medulla, the center of the brain that controls respiration."[37]

To treat alcoholism. In the nineteenth century U.S. doctors recommended cannabis as a treatment for delirium tremens. In 1953 Drs. L. Thompson and R. Proctor tested the synthetic cannabinoid Pyrahexyl in the treatment of alcohol withdrawal and obtained positive results in seventy cases.[38] In Jamaica and Costa Rica, where the use of ganja as an intoxicant is prevalent, the rate of alcoholism is much lower than elsewhere.[39]

To treat opiate addiction. In some cases, cannabis can serve to alleviate the symptoms of opiate withdrawal. As early as 1885, Dr. E. Birch reported the successful treatment of an opium addict and a chloral-hydrate addict by cannabis substitution followed by slow withdrawal of the cannabis.[40] In 1891 Dr. J. B. Mattison held that "it has proved an efficient substitute for the poppy," and described the case of a naval surgeon, "nine years a ten grains daily subcutaneous morphia taker . . . [who] recovered with less than a dozen doses."[41] He recommended cannabis as "a drug that has a special value in some morbid conditions, and the intrinsic merit and safety of which entitles it to a place it once held in therapeutics. . . . Indian hemp is not here lauded as a specific. It will, at times, fail. So do other drugs. But the many cases in which it acts well, entitle it to a large and lasting confidence."[42]

To alleviate insomnia. In 1890 the British physician J. Reynolds highly recommended *Cannabis indica* for patients having what was then called "senile insomnia." "In this class of cases," he said, "I have found nothing comparable in utility to a moderate dose of Indian hemp," which remains effective for years without producing

tolerance. CBD induces sleep in insomniacs with fewer dreams and no side effects.[43]

For relief from herpes. Although one report published in a major immunology journal indicated that THC reduces resistance to the herpes simplex virus,[44] a separate study has shown that THC binds to the herpes virus and thus inactivates it. Topical application of an isopropyl alcohol extract of cannabis has been used to provide symptomatic relief of herpes sores. It prevents blisters and makes sores disappear within a day. Cannabis also provides symptomatic relief from gonorrhea and syphillis.[45]

For relief from migraine. Cannabis was used regularly in the nineteenth century to provide relief from migraine headaches. In an 1887 issue of the *Therapeutic Gazette*, H. A. Hare testified to the value of hemp in subduing migraines and preventing further attacks.[46] In 1890 Dr. J. Reynolds noted in the *Lancet* that "many victims of this malady have for years kept their suffering in abeyance by taking hemp at the moment of threatening, or onset of the attack."[47] One year later Dr. J. B. Mattison asserted that, of all the applications of cannabis, "its most important use is in that opprobrium of the healing arts—

■■■

Joe Zias and colleagues found skeletal remains of a fourteen-year-old girl from the fourth century buried in a family tomb in Beit Shemesh, near Jerusalem, Israel in 1993. The archaeologists found the skeletal remains of a full-term fetus in the girl's pelvis, which was too small to allow the childbirth and caused her death by hemorrhage. Several grams of gray, carbonized matter recovered with the body proved to be cannabis. Perhaps it had been administered in an attempt to stop the uterine bleeding, was burnt for a ritual purpose, or was inhaled for analgesia.[48]

■■■

migraine," and he concluded that the drug not only stopped migraine headaches, but could also be used to prevent the attacks.[49] In *The Principles and Practice of Medicine* (1913), Dr. William Osler affirmed that "cannabis is probably the most satisfactory remedy" for migraines.[50]

For treatment of ulcer. Stomach-acid output decreases after the consumption of cannabis, which recommends it for the treatment of peptic ulcers, colitis, ileitis, spastic colon, and gastritis. Preparations of cannabis were used for those purposes in the 1890s.[51]

In gynecology. Cannabis has been used successfully in the treatment of hyperemesis gravidarum, a form of morning sickness in which the pregnant woman suffers from constant nausea and vomiting. Cannabis reduces pain and increases uterine contractions more quickly than ergot alkaloids. Native women in South Africa stupefy themselves with cannabis (called *dagga*) to facilitate delivery. Dr. J. Grigor rediscovered the oxytocic properties of Indian hemp in 1852, and stated more or less altruistically, "it is capable of bringing the labor to a happy conclusion considerably within half the time that would otherwise have been required, thus saving protracted suffering to

the patient, and the time of the practitioner."[52] Cannabis also is a valuable remedy in the treatment of mastitis, dysmenorrhea, menstrual and postpartum pain, and it has been used to increase lactation. Queen Victoria herself smoked cannabis to relieve her menstrual cramps.

In 1883, Dr. John Brown recommended the use of cannabis in uterine dysfunctions, asserting, "There is no medicine which has given such good results. . . . the failures are so few, that I venture to call it a specific in menorrhagia [excessive uterine bleeding]."[53] His fellow Dr. Robert Batho agreed: "Considerable experience of its employment in menorrhagia, more especially in India, has convinced me that it is, in that country at all events, one of the most reliable means at our disposal."[54]

Hemp Seed and Nutrition

Hemp seed has served as a primary famine food in China, Australia, and Europe as recently as World War II. Hemp seed is eaten today by many of India's poor people: a mixture called *bosa* consists of the seeds of goosegrass (eleusine) and hemp, and *mura* is

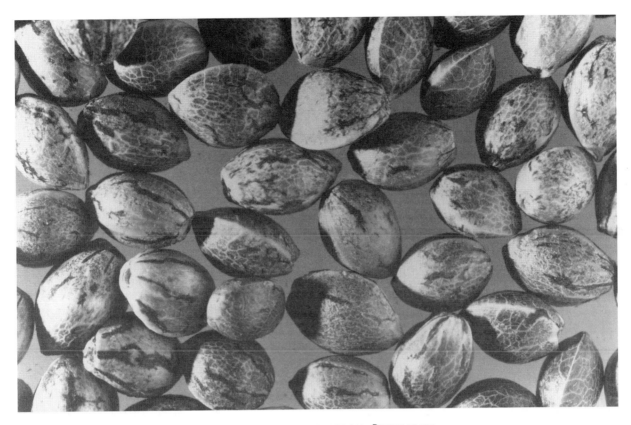

Hemp seed—the most complete protein in the vegetable kingdom. Photograph courtesy of the USDA.

made with parched wheat, amaranth or rice, and hemp seed. The seeds are said to make all vegetables more palatable and complete foods. Sometimes it is an ingredient in chutney. Bhang and ripe hemp seed also is used to flavor or strengthen the formulations of alcoholic beverages. And mothers of the Sotho tribe in South Africa are known to feed their babies with ground hemp seed in pap.[55]

Hemp seed contains all the essential amino acids and fatty acids, and is the most complete protein to be found in the vegetable kingdom. The seed contains 26 to 31 percent crude protein. The meal also contains about 6 percent carbohydrates, 5 to 10 percent fat, 12 percent crude fiber, 10 percent moisture, and 7 percent ash.[56]

The globulin edestin found in hemp protein closely resembles the globulin found in blood plasma, and it is easily digested,

---

···

Cannabis Cuisine

Over the centuries and across the continents, cannabis has been incorporated into the cooking of many cultures, and hundreds of recipes can be found or invented. The psychoactive cannabinoids are fat-soluble, and usually are extracted into clarified butter.

The acclaimed artist and chef Agmed Yacoubi, who makes the claim of being the direct descendant of the prophet Mohammed on both parents' sides, offers a guide to the ancient science of Moroccan cuisine in the *Alchemist's Cookbook* (1972), including some basic recipes using kif:

BHANG

Grind some kif leaves with equal amounts of black pepper, cloves, nutmeg, and mace. Mix with a little water, then strain. Mix with water, milk, watermelon juice, or cucumber juice.

Bhang is often drunk without the spices, but the spices are believed to make it more powerful.

···

···

Hemp Seed Tahini
(pure ground hemp seed)

Nutrition Facts
Serving Size: 2 Tbsp (32g)

Calories: 160

	% Daily Value*
Total Fat 9g	14%
Saturated Fat 0g	0%
Cholesterol 0mg	0%
Total Carbohydrate 11g	3%
Dietary Fiber 11g	45%
Sugars 0g	
Protein 8g	25%

Vitamin A 24% • Riboflavin 21%

Thiamine 25% • Niacin 4%

*Percent Daily Values are based on a 2000 calorie diet

···

---

absorbed, and utilized by the human body. It is vital to the maintenance of a healthy immune system, being used to manufacture antibodies against invasive agents.[57] Scientists have been studying the use of hemp seed extracts to boost the immune systems of individuals with AIDS and cancer.

Hemp edestin is so compatible with the human digestive system that the Czechoslovakian Tubercular Nutrition Study conducted in 1955 found hemp seed to be the only food that can successfully treat the consumptive disease tuberculosis, in which the nutritive processes are impaired and the body wastes away.[58] Edestin is considered such a perfect protein that in 1941 *Science* complained that "Passage of the Marijuana Law of 1937 has placed restrictions upon trade in hempseed that, in effect, amount to prohibition. . . . It seems clear that the long and important career of the protein is coming to a close in the United States."[59]

Hemp seed's weight is 30 to 35 percent oil, 80 percent of which consists of the unsaturated essential fatty acids (EFAs) linoleic acid and linolenic acid, which are not manufactured by the body and must be supplied by food. The oil also contains about 8 percent by volume of palmitic, stearic, oleic, and arachidic acids. The 80 percent EFAs in hemp-seed oil is the highest total percentage among the common plants used by man. Flax oil ranks second with 72 percent EFAs. The EFAs are very sensitive to heat, light, and oxygen; thus, hemp-seed oil must be processed and stored carefully (in the cold and dark, and under vacuum) to preserve the potency of the EFAs.

EFAs are precursors to the prostaglandin series (PGE 1, 2, and 3). PGE 1 inhibits the production of cholesterol and dilates blood vessels, and it prevents the clotting of blood platelets in arteries. A study reported in 1992 indicated that a diet of hemp seed causes the serum levels of total cholesterol to drop dramatically.[60] Blood pressure also decreases after several weeks of eating hemp seed, apparently due to the steady supply of EFAs.[61]

Veterinary Uses

Cannabis has been widely used in Asia to treat the diseases of animals. It is commonly fed to elephants and oxen to relieve their fatigue and give them greater endurance and strength. Wild hemp leaves are burned in heaps to disinfect stables and barns and to treat respiratory problems. A bolus of hemp flowers, sugar, and grain is fed to livestock to treat colic, constipation, diarrhea, worms, and rinderpest (a form of diptheria). Bhang is fed to cattle before mating and to increase lactation.

When hemp seed is fed to poultry on a regular basis, the birds do not go "off feed," and they do not require hormones to fatten them. Egg production also is increased. Hemp seed meal has an effect analogous to that of grit in chicken diets, keeping their gizzard linings free of corrugations and erosions.[62]

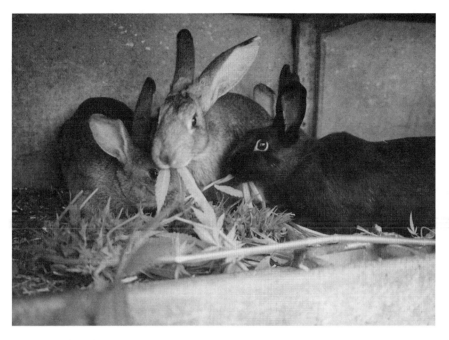

HEMP IS A WELCOME PART OF THE DIET OF MANY SPECIES. PHOTOGRAPH COURTESY OF SWIHTCO.

Public Health Studies around the World

Perhaps more than any plant used by man, hemp has been subject to a barrage of studies. The majority of these studies have attempted to "convict" hemp of some of the accusations directed toward it in the last century, particularly the question of whether it causes moral or physical decline. As Lester Grinspoon of Harvard Medical School puts it, "This vast research enterprise has completely failed to provide a scientific basis

■■■

U. Erasmus, author of *Fats That Heal, Fats That Kill*, believes that the proportions of linoleic and linolenic acid in hemp seed oil are perfectly balanced to meet human requirements for EFAs. Unlike flax oil and others, hemp-seed oil can be used continuously without developing either a deficiency or imbalance of EFAs. In addition, the peroxide value (PV)—the degree of rancidity—of hemp-seed oil is 0.1 to 0.5, which is very low and safe and does not spoil its taste. In comparison, the PV of virgin olive oil is about 20, and the PV of corn oil is about 40 to 60.[63]

■■■

for prohibition."[64] Remarkably, the millions of dollars world governments have thrown into their war on hemp have backfired; these studies now provide some of the best evidence of the myriad benefits of hemp, and several have recommended its legalization.

The Indian Hemp Drugs Commission (1893–94). In the 1870s government officials in India commonly blamed ganja as a cause of insanity and crime, since users of ganja were poor, helpless, and convenient scapegoats. English bureaucrats were complaining about ganja abuse, and in 1893 Lord Kimberly, India's secretary of state, appointed the Indian Hemp Drugs Commission.[65]

The seven commissioners (four English, three Indian, including a raja) interviewed 1193 witnesses between August 1893 and August 1894. The commissioners concluded that "the occasional use of hemp in moderate doses may be beneficial; but this use may be regarded as medicinal in character." The commission was of the opinion that moderate use of hemp had "no evil results at all." Addresssing the concerns that had been raised about ganja use, they maintained that it caused no appreciable physical injury of any kind, no injurious effects on the mind, and no moral injury whatever. The commission warned against the consequences of excessive use, noting that "as in the case of other intoxicants, excessive use tends to weaken the constitution and to render the consumer more susceptible to disease. . . . Excessive use of hemp drugs may, especially in cases where there is any weakness or hereditary predisposition, induce insanity." But, the report continued, "It has been shown that the effect of hemp drugs in this respect has hitherto been greatly exaggerated."

The Commission decided that "total prohibition of the cultivation of the hemp plant for narcotics, and of the manufacture, sale, or use of the drugs derived from it is neither necessary nor expedient in consideration of their ascertained effects, of the prevalence of the habit of using them, of the social and religious feeling on the subject, and of the possibility of its driving the consumers to have recourse to other stimulants or narcotics which may be more deleterious."[66]

The Canal Zone Studies. The Republic of Panama prohibited the "cultivation, use, and consumption of the herb Kan-Jac [cannabis]" in 1923 just as concern about reports of American soldiers smoking cannabis prompted the provost marshall to prohibit its possession by military personnel in the Canal Zone. A formal committee was convened in April 1925 to investigate the use of marijuana. The committee, which was chaired by Colonel J. F. Siler of the Army Medical Corps, observed some soldiers, four doctors, and two police officers smoking cannabis without untoward effect. A lieutenant on the committee declared:

> I think we can safely say, based upon samples we have smoked here and upon the reports of the individuals concerned, that there is nothing to indicate any habit forming tendency or any striking ill effects. All of the statements to the effect that two or three puffs produce remarkable effects are nonsense, judging from our experience.

The committee concluded that cannabis was not addictive and did not have "any appreciable deleterious influence on the individuals using it." Some commanders disagreed with the committee's findings and ordered a new investigation in 1929. The surgeon general who directed the inquiry duly reported that "use of the drug is not widespread and . . . its effects upon military efficiency and upon discipline are not

great." A third investigation, initiated in June 1931, found no link between cannabis and delinquency or morale problems.[67]

The LaGuardia Committee Report. In 1938 the Mayor of New York, Frank H. LaGuardia, requested that the New York Academy of Medicine appoint a special subcommittee to study cannabis. Subsequently, in 1944 the Committee on Marihuana published its report, *The Marihuana Problem in the City of New York.* The study comprised sociological, clinical, and pharmacological studies. The clinical study considered medical aspects (symptoms, systemic functions, addiction, tolerance, and possible therapeutic applications), psychological and intellectual functioning, emotional reactions, general personality structure, and family and community ideologies. The committee refuted all the derogatory claims made against cannabis, and made the following conclusions:

- "The consensus among marihuana smokers is that the use of the drug creates a feeling of adequacy."
- "The practice of smoking marihuana does not lead to addiction in the medical sense of the word."
- "The use of marihuana does

not lead to morphine or heroin or cocaine addiction and no effort is made to create a market for these narcotics by stimulating the practice of marihuana smoking."

- "Marihuana is not the determining factor in the commission of major crimes."
- "The publicity concerning the catastrophic effects of marihuana smoking in New York City is unfounded."[69]

The Wooton Report. The British Advisory Committee on Drug Dependence appointed the Hallucinogens Sub-Committee, chaired by Baroness Barbara Wooton, to review the literary evidence about cannabis. The 1968 Wooton Report on Cannabis confirmed earlier studies:

> Having reviewed all the material available to us we find ourselves in agreement with the conclusion reached by the Indian Hemp Drugs Commission appointed by the Government of India (1893–1894) and the New York Mayor's Committee on Marihuana (1944) that the long-term consumption of cannabis in moderate doses has no harmful effects.[70]

The Shafer Commission. The Comprehensive Drug Abuse Prevention and Control Act of 1970 also established the National Commission on Cannabis and Drug Abuse, chaired by former Pennsylvania governor Raymond Shafer. That commission concluded:

> There is no evidence that experimental or intermittent use of marihuana causes physical or psychological harm. The risk lies instead in heavy, long-term use of the drug. Marihuana does not lead to physical dependency, although some evidence indicates that heavy, long-term users may develop a psychological dependence on the drug.

The Shafer Commission tried to put to rest several other issues feeding public anxiety about the results of cannabis use, concluding that "Psychosis resulting from marihuana use is extremely rare and such reactions tend to occur in predisposed individuals," and that "the present level of marihuana use in American society does not constitute a threat to the public health." Contrary to government propaganda, "The overwhelming majority of marihuana users do not progress to drugs other than alcohol," although "Statistically marihuana users are more likely to experiment with other drugs than are non-users."[71]

■■■

The LaGuardia Committee tested for alterations in subjects' family values and ideologies under the influence of cannabis. Their results? It was found that "the only very definite change as a result of the ingestion of marihuana was in their attitude toward the drug itself. Without marihuana only 4 out of 14 subjects said they would tolerate the sale of marihuana, while after ingestion 8 of them were in favor of this."[68]

■■■

The Jamaica Study. In 1970 the National Institute of Mental Health's Center for Studies of Narcotic and Drug Abuse sponsored the Jamaica Study, a project in medical anthropology that became "the first intensive, multidisciplinary study of cannabis use and users to be published."[72]

The Jamaica Study staff examined the legislation, ethnohistory, and social complex of ganja, and the acute effects of smoking in a natural setting. Clinical studies evaluated respiratory function and hematology, electroencephalography, and psychiatric condition, and psychological assessments were made of the seventy subjects. The complex ganja culture from which the subjects were drawn pervades and greatly influences the working-class community. In some communities, 50 percent of the males over the age of fifteen smoked ganja regularly, and only 20 percent were absolute nonsmokers.

The foreword to Vera Rubin and Lambros Comitas's 1975 report, *Ganja in Jamaica,* was written by Raymond Shafer and is worth reproducing at length:

While Americans are concerned with the alleged "amotivational" and drug-escalation effects of marihuana, ganja in Jamaica serves to fulfill values of the work ethic; for example, the primary use of ganja by working-class males is as an energizer. Furthermore, there is no problem of drug escalation in the Jamaican working class; as a multipurpose plant, ganja is used medicinally, even by nonsmokers, and is taken in teas by women and children for prophylactic and therapeutic purposes. For such users, there is no reliance even on patent medicines, amphetamines, or barbiturates, let alone heroin and LSD. Further, the use of ganja appears to be a "benevolent alternative" to heavy consumption of alcohol by the working class. Admissions to the mental hospital in Jamaica for alcoholism account for less than 1 percent annually, in contrast to other Caribbean areas where ganja use is not pervasive and admission rates for alcoholism are as high as 55 percent.

This study indicates that there is little correlation between use of ganja and crime, except insofar as the possession and cultivation of ganja are technically crimes. There were no indications of organic brain damage or chromosome damage among the subjects and no significant clinical (psychiatric, psychological or medical) differences between the smokers and controls. . . .

Despite its illegality, ganja use is

■■■
Cannabis Linguistics

Marijuana—the dried leaves, and sometimes flowers, of the hemp plant. Usually smoked in a cigarette.

Bhang—the Hindu equivalent of marijuana. Also refers to a liquid mixture of hemp leaves, milk, sugar, and spices. Drunk in India, particularly on Shiva's birthday.

Ganja—the dried flowering tops of the female hemp plant. More powerful than bhang.

Hashish—the dried resin produced by the female hemp plant. Can be smoked or eaten. Contains the most THC of any hemp preparation.

Charas—Indian word for hashish.

Kif—the Arabic word for hemp preparations.

Dagga—South African term for dried hemp preparations.

Cannabis—short for *Cannabis sativa* L., or *Cannabis indica*. Often used to distinguish the dried, psychoactive *cannabis* preparations from the living *hemp* plant.

■■■

pervasive, and duration and frequency are very high; it is smoked over a longer period in greater quantities with greater THC potency than in the United States, without deleterious social or psychological consequences. The major difference is that both ganja use and expected behaviors are culturally conditioned and controlled by well-established tradition. The findings throw new light on the cannabis question, particularly that the relationship between man and marihuana is not simply pharmaceutical, and indicate the need for new approaches.[73]

The Jamaica Study also afforded due respect to the Rastafari religion, in which ganja is regarded as a sacrament and a gift of God:

Ganja, unlike alcohol, has special symbolic attributes. Rastafarian metaphysics, for example, emphasizes and brings into focus general concepts derived from working-class views of ganja. For them, it is "the wisdom weed," of divine origin, an elixir vitae, documented by Biblical chapter and verse which overrides man-made proscriptions. Religious authority thus validates and fortifies commitment to its use; there is no need to invoke religious validations of alcohol consumption, which is legally and socially accepted. While drinking in the local bar may enhance feelings of sociability, the sacred source of ganja permits a sense of religious communication, marked by meditation and contemplation.[74]

Melanie Dreher, an anthropologist at the University of Miami, was a key member of the Jamaica team. In a subsequent study, *Working Men and Ganja,* she reported that the drinking of ganja tea or tonic extracts is widespread in Jamaica, even by nonsmokers and children. "The health-rendering effects of these preparations are reported for a wide variety of general and specific disorders," she found. "Ganja poultices and compresses are used . . . for the relief of pain, open wounds, and skin eruptions."[75]

The Jamaica Study was good science: rigorous, controlled, and well supported. So why was it not more influential? According to Dreher, members of a presidential commission told her they weren't interested in the results of her work if it failed to show negative effects of cannabis use.

The Costa Rica Study. In 1971 the University of Florida and the National Institutes of Health cooperated in a study led by William Carter to examine chronic cannabis use in Costa Rica. Eighty-four cannabis smokers and 156 control subjects who had never smoked ganja underwent a battery of sophisticated medical and psychological examinations. The results were equivalent to those of the Jamaica study, with few notable differences: the similarities outweighed the differences between users and nonusers, and ganja smokers generally enjoyed longer-lasting relationships with their mates. The Costa Rica study also found no significant health consequences to chronic cannabis smokers.[76]

The NIH refused to accept the report for publication, demanding that it be rewritten three times. Still not satisfied, the NIH then had it rewritten by another editor and ultimately printed only three hundred copies. A copy of the original version was leaked to the National Organization for the Reform of Marijuana Laws.[77]

The Greek Study. In a 1975 study of hashish smokers in Greece, C. N. Stefanis and M. R. Issodorides presented microphotographs of damaged human sperm and suggested that the low arginine content in the sperm nuclei indicated "deviant maturation." It was later revealed, however, that the photographs had been doctored, and Stefanis and

Issodorides were obliged to issue a "correction of misinformation" in the journal *Science.* The major finding of the "Greek study," which had been sponsored by the U.S. Government's National Institute on Drug Abuse, was that even after twenty-five years of use, the acute effects of hashish appeared to be qualitatively similar to the effects on less experienced users.[78]

The Coptic Study. A 1981 study by two UCLA psychologists tested the physical and mental health of ten members of the Jamaica-based Ethiopian Zion Coptic Church. Like Rastafarians, the Zion Coptics believe the use of ganja to be "a spiritual, integral act" and they claim, for example, that the burning bush in the epic of Moses symbolized cannabis. The church has official recognition as an organized religion by the government of Jamaica and the Supreme Court of Florida. The study showed that the IQs of Zion Coptics actually increased after they began to use ganja.[79]

The Expert Group. The British Advisory Council on the Misuse of Drugs released the *Report of the Expert Group on the Effects of Cannabis Use* in 1982, which stated that "there is insufficient evidence to enable us to reach incontestable conclusions as to the effects

The U.S. Government's response to the overwhelming evidence from studies indicating the beneficial qualities of cannabis is typified by James O. Mason, head of the U.S. Public Health Service. Mason administered the IND program, which provided legal cannabis to an experimental group of patients with AIDS or cancer. In 1991 requests for cannabis from people with AIDS exploded; instead of expanding the program, Mason canceled it. His rationale: "If it is perceived that the Public Health Service is going around giving marijuana to folks, there would be a perception that this stuff can't be so bad."[80]

on the human body of the use of cannabis." With seeming trepidation the report concluded, "There is evidence to suggest that the therapeutic use of cannabis or of substances derived from it for the treatment of certain medical conditions may, after further research, prove to be beneficial."[81]

Physical and Mental Effects of Hemp

PHYSICAL EFFECTS

Heavy smoking of cannabis (several times daily) causes mild constriction of airways. Light smoking of cannabis has little effect on breathing, except for bronchodilation. Ventilatory mechanics and gas exchange remain normal, except for a transient stimulatory effect on oxygen consumption and CO_2 ventilation. THC is not a respiratory depressant. Chronic smoking can produce inflammation, sinusitis, pharyngitis, bronchitis, and coughing of sputum. Decrease of consumption provides relief, but antibiotics do not. Cannabis decreases the salivary flow in the submaxillary gland, resulting in a dry mouth.[82]

There is scant evidence of a direct carcinogenic effect of cannabis smoke or tar. Some experiments with cannabis tar have produced mutations in several strains of bacteria, and rats painted with the tar have developed benign skin tumors. Cannabis smoke has been found to contain many of the same carcinogenic compounds as tobacco, but to date there have been no cases of cancer attributed to smoking cannabis. The effect of cannabis seems to accelerate, rather than initiate, malignant changes. The traditional water pipe serves well to mitigate the irritating effects of cannabis smoke.[83]

The most evident and immediate effect of smoking or ingesting cannabis is a rapid increase in heart rate (up to ninety beats per minute), which diminishes within an hour and poses no threat to a healthy individual. Blood pressure may rise slightly, and postural hypotension can occur. Smokers develop a tolerance to the cardiac and psychotropic effects of THC after two to three weeks of daily smoking. Persons with vascular disease are at risk, however, and should not compromise their health with cannabis use. In a case reported in 1979, a twenty-five-year-old man developed an acute subendocardial infarction after smoking cannabis.[84]

Hypothermia. THC produces hypothermia (lower body temperature) in animals, but experiments with humans have shown little or no such effect except at high doses. Instead, skin temperature, metabolic rate, and heart rate are increased, but core temperature remains unchanged. Cannabis also inhibits sweating.[85]

Toxicity. Cannabis is nontoxic. No deaths from an overdose of cannabis have ever been verified; where a few poorly documented reports have given cannabis as the cause of death, closer examination has shown the accusations to be untenable. A few near-fatal intravenous injections of a water extract of cannabis have been reported.[86]

It has been estimated that one would have to smoke eight hundred cannabis cigarettes to induce a fatal reaction, and even then one would probably receive a lethal dose of carbon monoxide first. In comparison, only sixty milligrams of nicotine or three hundred milliliters of alcohol can be fatal.[87]

Effect on male reproduction. After numerous experiments, it has been determined that THC produces a mild, reversible suppressive effect on sperm production, but does not seem to have any negative effect on male fertility.[88] A few cases of "pubertal arrest" have been reported, such as the instance of a seventeen-year-old male who had smoked cannabis several times daily since age eleven and still had not attained puberty. After a few months of abstinence from cannabis, his growth accelerated, his genital enlarged, and his levels of testosterone and luteinizing hormone rose.

A 1974 study led by R. Kolodny reported that the plasma testosterone, luteinizing hormone (LH), follicle-stimulating hormone (FSH), prolactin levels, and sperm counts of twenty men who regularly smoked cannabis were significantly lower than controls. The report sparked a controversy that has smoldered for years. Other researchers later concluded that the observed short-term effects are caused by direct action upon the seminiferous tubular epithelium of the testes. The accumulated research offers potential for the development of a male chemical contraceptive.[89]

Gynecomastia. The enlargement of breast glands in males, a common transient occurrence among adolescents, has long been rumored to be affected by cannabis use. Gynecomastia also is caused by cirrhosis of the liver, by testicular, adrenal, and pituitary tumors, and by steroids, amphetamines, and other drugs. In 1972 a team of researchers presented

A recent study of Jamaican infants found that at one month of age children of cannabis-smoking mothers scored significantly higher than children born to non-smokers in ten of the fourteen characteristics measured, including alertness, robustness, regulatory capacity, and orientation. The mothers reported that cannabis increased their appetites, relieved their morning sickness, and improved the quality of their rest. These effects likely contributed to the healthier newborns.[90]

fourteen cases of breast development in young men who had smoked cannabis for several years. Other causes were excluded. Only three of the fourteen patients experienced a decrease in breast development after abstaining from cannabis. A controlled study in 1977 of eleven gynecomastic U.S. soldiers in Germany found only "a non-association between idiopathic gynecomastia and chronic cannabis use." If cannabis has any effect on gynecomastia, it depends on dosage, potency, frequency of use, and the endocrinology of the individual.[91]

Effect on female reproduction. Experiments with rats have demonstrated some teratogenic effects (malformations) and decreased conception caused by cannabis, but the results are considered to be of only marginal relevance to humans, because the route of administration, solvent medium, concentration, and high dosage are extremely unnatural and unrealistic. Insulin, penicillin, cortisone and aspirin produce the same effects. The Relman Committee report *Marihuana and Health* concluded that despite widespread cannabis use by young women of reproductive age, "there is no evidence yet of any teratogenic effects of high frequency or consistent association with the

drug." The committee knew of isolated reports of congenital anomalies in the offspring of cannabis users, but had not seen evidence that they occurred more often in users than in nonusers.[92]

Johnathan Buckley, however, conducted a case-control study of in-utero exposure to cannabis and reported a possible link between maternal use of mind altering drugs prior to and during pregnancy and an increase in the risk of acute non-lymphocytic leukemia (ANLL) in offspring. "Although the association of marihuana exposure in utero and subsequent development of ANLL has not been firmly established," the study reported, "the evidence is strong enough to justify further study." In one report babies born to marijuana-smoking mothers were shorter, weighed less, had smaller heads, and cried less at birth.[93]

Cerebral Atrophy. In the 1970s considerable controversy was generated by sensational reports alleging that smoking cannabis caused "brain damage." The only two studies that were able to produce results to corroborate these allegations are notable for their shockingly poor methodology. One study involved animals forced to smoke large amounts of cannabis in a few minutes through a smoking machine, without any opportunity to breathe normally. The animals were suffocated with the smoke. One can only assume that these researchers were aware that oxygen starvation is a reliable cause of brain damage.[94]

The second study, published in *The Lancet* in 1971, reported that the brains of ten heavy cannabis smokers showed signs of cerebral atrophy. The results were put in a questionable light, to say nothing of the scientists, once it became clear that up to half the subjects were schizophrenic, three had suffered head injuries, one was mentally retarded, one or two were epileptic, and *all ten* were culled from a psychiatric clinic. In addition, all had histories of abuse of LSD, opiates, tranquilizers, and other drugs.[95]

The Relman Committee report, *Marijuana and Health,* summarized the issue:

> There is substantial controversy about whether cannabis causes changes in brain structure or in brain cells. Two studies have reported that cannabis produces changes in brain morphology. Both suffer sufficiently from methodological and interpretational defects that their conclusions cannot be accepted. Furthermore, other studies have not found changes in morphology . . . There is no persuasive evidence that cannabis causes morphological changes in the brain. Computer tomography studies on users of cannabis reveal no gross changes in brain structure. Electron micrographic studies of monkey brains indicating morphologic changes are methodologically flawed and cannot be used as evidence for an effect of cannabis on brain cell morphology.[96]

MENTAL EFFECTS

Cannabis produces a wide spectrum of perceptual effects. These include mood changes, facilitation of interpersonal behavior, and reduction of aggressive behavior. In other words, cannabis usually makes people feel happy, sociable, and peaceful. Charles Tart has recorded a variety of perceptual phenomena that result from cannabis intoxication. Characteristic visual perceptions include patterns, vivid imagery, and improved peripheral vision. Hallucinations, auras, and dimensional changes occur less often. The senses of taste, smell, touch, and hearing are augmented with new qualities and greater intensity. Cannabis intoxication often creates a craving for sweets. The sense of time is consistently distorted by cannabis;

The most memorable case on record of a cannabis-induced panic attack involves an episode in which a Hindu man who smoked ganja for the first time experienced extreme depersonalization and could not feel his legs:

He then tried to feel the presence of his legs by deep pressure with his fingers, and to his utter surprise and horror he discovered that his penis had seemingly gone inside the abdomen beyond grasping or holding. At this feeling of "penis loss" he shouted for help. . . . His friends came hurriedly and "dragged out" the receded penis manually. He was in a state of acute psychogenic shock. . . . He was taken to a nearby pond with his penis held by one of his friends and he was put into the water . . . Eventually the victim perceived that the retracting penis had become stable and regained its usual morphology.[97]

events seem to last much longer than they really do. Another common effect is a strong sense of being "here-and-now." The phenomenon of deja vu often occurs. Ostensible paranormal phenomena such as empathy, intuition, or telepathy, as well as mystical experiences, often are reported. Cannabis is considered to be an aphrodisiac. Emotions are felt more strongly. Users often report that cannabis makes them feel more childlike and open to experience.[98]

Adverse Effects. As many as a third of regular cannabis users occasionally experience paranoid or panic reactions, hallucinations, confusion, and other adverse reactions, usually only in unfavorable settings and at high doses. The problem occurs most often when cannabis is ingested, apparently because the dose is not as easily controlled as with smoking. Medical treatment is rarely sought because the situation is easily self-controlled in most cases.

The so-called "acute brain syndrome," or delerium, attributed to cannabis abuse is distinguished by mental clouding, perceptual disturbances, disorientation, impaired goal-directed thinking and behavior, memory disorders, disruption of sleep patterns, and changes in psychomotor control. The symp-

toms develop quickly and fluctuate rapidly. The syndrome manifests during drug use and soon disappears with abstinence. Most of the reported cases have come from India and the Middle East, where the potency of cannabis products is generally higher and consumption is more widespread than in Europe and America. Cases have been reported among American soldiers in Vietnam and in Europe; the men recovered in three to eleven days and returned to duty.[99]

Learning. While cannabis may improve empathetic and conceptual receptivity, rote learning certainly suffers. Recall usually is impaired, apparently because of poor concentration. Numerous tests have shown that cannabis has adverse effects on short-term memory, persisting for two to three hours or longer.[100]

Dependence. The Merck Manual of Diagnosis and Therapy (1987) states that:

chronic or periodic administration of cannabis or cannabis substances produces some psychic dependence because of the desired subjective effects, but no physical dependence; there is no abstinence syndrome when the drug is discontinued.

Cannabis can be used on an episodic but continual basis without evidence of social or psychic dysfunction. In many users the term dependence with its obvious connotations probably is misapplied. . . . The chief opposition to the drug rests on a moral and political, and not a toxicologic, foundation.[101]

It is worth noting that so pervasive was the stigma against cannabis at the height of Ronald Reagan's "Zero Tolerance" policy that the *Merck Manual* felt it necessary to qualify their scientific findings.

Psychological Health. In 1990 J. Shedler and J. Block published the results of a rigorous study of 101 youths whom they had followed from age 3 to 23, examining their psychological health in relation to drug use. The researchers found that adolescents who had experimented occasionally with drugs, particularly with cannabis, were well adjusted, while

adolescents who used drugs frequently were maladjusted, showing a distinct personality syndrome marked by interpersonal alienation, poor impulse control, and manifest emotional distress. Adolescents who had never experimented with any drug were relatively anxious, emotionally constricted, and lacking in social

skills. Psychological differences between frequent drug users, experimenters, and abstainers could be traced to the earliest years of childhood and related to the quality of their parenting. The findings indicate that (a) problem drug use is a symptom, not a cause, of personal and social maladjustment, and (b) the meaning of drug use can be understood only in the context of an individual's personality structure and developmental history. . . . Current efforts at drug "education" seem flawed on two counts. First, they are alarmist, pathologizing normative adolescent experimentation . . . and perhaps frightening parents and educators unnecessarily. Second, and of far greater concern, they trivialize the factors underlying drug abuse, implicitly denying their depth and pervasiveness.[102]

"It's absolutely not the case that experimentation leads to abuse," says Johnathan Shedler, co-author of a study indicating that youths who become addicts share three psychological factors that make them susceptible: "poor impulse control; unhappiness—they were anxious, distressed or depressed; and alienation—they had few friends, they weren't invested in anything like sports or family relations." Psychologist

Judith Brook concluded from similar studies that "parental support, warmth, responsiveness, affection, and the child's identification with the parent" were fundamental to prevention of drug abuse in later years. Yet another study also refuted the association of cannabis with amotivation, instead finding that poly-drug use (including alcohol, amphetamines, and cocaine) seemed more associated with the syndrome.[103]

In one comparison of cannabis users and nonusers, individuals who did not smoke cannabis scored slightly higher on psychological tests for sociability, communality, responsibility, and achievement by conformity, partly because they were "too deferential to external authority, narrow in their interests and over-controlled." Cannabis smokers scored higher for empathy and independent achievement, and had better social perception and more sensitivity to the feelings and needs of others. The researchers concluded that cannabis smokers possess all the "achievement motivation necessary for success in graduate school."[104]

Amotivational syndrome. Some chronic users of cannabis exhibit a group of personality changes that clinicians are wont to call "amotivational syndrome." The changes include apathy, loss of ambition and energy, poor concentration, and a decline in work or scholastic performance. The issue of "amotivational syndrome" largely began in 1971, when the *Journal of the American Medical Association* published an article entitled "Effects of Marihuana on Adolescents and Young Adults" by Harold Kolansky and William Moore. The pair described thirty-eight cannabis smokers, thirteen to twenty-four years old, who "showed an onset of psychiatric problems shortly after the beginning of marihuana smoking; these individuals had either no premorbid psychiatric history or had premorbid psychiatric symptoms which were extremely mild or almost unnoticeable in contrast to the serious symptomatology which followed the known onset of marihuana smoking."[105] Although the authors could show an association between smoking cannabis and mental problems, they did not demonstrate a causal relationship, nor did they explain the mechanism of "ego decompensation," which they repeatedly stated was due to the "toxic" effect of cannabis. The unqualified report generated a storm of controversy. Lester Grinspoon considered Kolansky and Moore's report to be irresponsible.

All in all this paper is, from a scientific point of view, so unsound as to be all but meaningless. Unfortunately, from a social point of view it will have a great significance in that it confirms for those people who have a hyperemotional bias against cannabis all the things they would like to believe happen as a consequence of the use of cannabis and in turn it will enlarge the credibility gap which exists between young people and the medical profession. I am convinced that if the American Medical Association were less interested in the imposition of a moral hegemony with respect to this issue and more concerned with the scientific aspects of this drug this paper would not have been accepted for publication.[106]

Contrary to Kolansky and Moore, the Jamaica Study found that ganja enabled people to work harder, faster, and longer: "For energy, ganja is taken in the morning, during breaks in the work routine, or immediately before particularly onerous work. . . . the effects of small doses of ganja in the natural setting are negligible, while concentration on the work task itself increases markedly after smoking." The Jamaica researchers asserted that "the belief that ganja acts as a work stimulant and the behavior that this induces casts considerable doubt on the universality of what has been described in the literature as 'the amotivational syndrome.'" They quoted Dr. Andrew Weil, who suggests that in the United States "amotivation [is] a cause of heavy marihuana smoking rather than the reverse."[107]

What are we to make of claims that the same substance causes animals and Jamaican laborers to work harder but causes American adolescents to lose energy and ambition? Perhaps the two effects aren't as mutually exclusive as they at first seem. The key lies in the twentieth century's interpretation of "amotivational," and in cannabis's famous psychoactive ability to suspend time. Contentment in the current moment, the "here-and-now," helps ease the tedium of a Jamaican's physical labor, but that same here-and-now mentality is deadly to the modern Church of Progress, which preaches survival-of-the-fittest competition, and motivates through the promise of material wealth. Hemp's enhancement of the current moment, and of empathy and independent thinking, throws this whole ideology into question. Why devote endless hours to accumulating wealth to buy a happiness and satisfaction that already thrives within each and every moment? Doubts about the wisdom of twentieth-century motivations becomes "amotivational syndrome." In this sense hemp is a very real threat to modern culture, and it is no wonder that it has been targeted for extermination by the corporate world and its government allies.

Neurology

The discovery of receptors in the human brain specifically designed for cannabinoids should end the debate on their appropriateness for human beings. The receptor site, a protein on the cell surface, activates G-proteins inside the cell and leads to a cascade of other biochemical reactions that generate euphoria.[108]

In 1984 Miles Herkenham and his colleagues at the National Institute of Mental Health mapped cannabis's receptors in the brain, using radioactivated analogs of THC developed by Pfizer Central Research. They found the most receptors in the hippocampus, where memory consolidation occurs and where we translate the external world into a cognitive and spatial "map," and in the ce-rebral cortex, where higher cognition is performed. Very few receptors are found in the brain-stem, where the automatic life-support systems are controlled.[109] This may explain why it is virtually impossible to die from an overdose of cannabis. The presence of THC receptors in the basal ganglia—an area of the brain involved in the coordination of movement—may enable the cannabinoids to relieve spasticity. Some receptors are located in the spinal cord, and may be the site of the analgesic activity of cannabis. A few receptors are found in the testes, possibly accounting for the effects of THC on spermatogenesis and the sex drive.[110]

In 1992 William Devane identified a cannabinoid-like neurotransmitter produced by the human brain having biological and behavioral effects similar to THC. He named it anandamide, after the Sanskrit word *ananda,* meaning bliss.[111] The importance of these discoveries cannot be overstated. We now have scientific evidence for what so many world cultures have known all along: that only a handful of plants on Earth are welcomed as naturally by the human mind as is hemp. The concentration of cannabinoid receptors in the areas of the brain devoted to the higher mental processes—

memory, cognition, creativity—is striking. Hemp seems custom designed to sustain our soul as well as our body. Is it chance, then, that hemp's first appearance on the world stage, ten thousand years ago, coincided with man's first explosion of creativity in the form of the first civilizations? Or was that first tickle of cannabis on our infant imaginations the missing ingredient in the awakening of our higher mind?

Whether by design or coincidence, the bond between hemp and mankind is an ancient one. We have relied on this plant to feed, clothe, stimulate, and heal, and the relationship has proven as fruitful as that between human and canine. And just as man's best friend has moved from the forests and savannahs to a spot at the family hearth, after ten thousand years of service hemp has earned a trusted place in our homes.

3

HEMP
AND
SPIRITUALITY

Hemp and Human Consciousness

Terence McKenna credits psychotropic plants like cannabis with many of the qualities more conventional spiritual advocates assign to God. McKenna, a cultivator of shamanic plants and today's leading proponent of the psychedelic experience, theorizes that hallucinogenic plants are the medium of a massive transfer of information from the vegetable kingdom to the human species. He writes, "All of the mental functions which we associate with humanness, including recall, projective imagination, language, naming, magical speech, dance, and a sense of *religio* may have emerged out of interaction with hallucinogenic plants."[1]

Intriguing as his vision may be, you don't have to buy McKenna's ideas wholesale to trace a spiritual partnership between humans and hemp going back ten thousand years, when Old World hunter-gatherers made the transition to agriculture. Scholars commonly name hemp as one of the first agricultural crops, but science writer Carl Sagan suggests that its use for altering consciousness may be older still. In *The Dragons of Eden* Sagan notes that, according to a friend who has visited with the tribe, the hunter-gatherer Pygmies intoxicate themselves with marihuana before stalking their game, the better to endure the drudgery. The plant is their only cultivated crop, which they say they have used since the

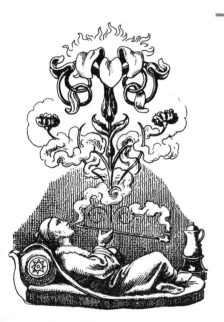

AN 1843 HASHISH SMOKER FROM M. VON SCHWIND'S *ALBUM OF ETCHINGS.*

74

dawn of time. "It would be wryly interesting," says Sagan, "if in human history the cultivation of marihuana led generally to the invention of agriculture, and thereby to civilization."[2]

Like both McKenna and Sagan, many historians assume that the effect of cannabis on consciousness was discovered soon after early humans discovered the plant itself. Archaic peoples freely sampled plants in their environment as possible food sources. Thus, they would have soon detected that this fast-growing weed fed more than their bellies.

But more than happy accidents may explain hemp's sacred role. Many religious scholars suggest that the ancients would naturally have expected plants to hold the secrets of the heavens. Plants draw nourishment from both moisture above and soil below. As such, our predecessors may have viewed them as obvious intermediaries between heaven and earth and thus the perfect key to the divine mysteries. And because of hemp's multitude of practical uses, the ancients might have looked to it first.

As discussed in the previous chapter, almost five thousand years ago the Chinese emperor Shen Nung recommended hemp as a remedy for malaria, constipa-

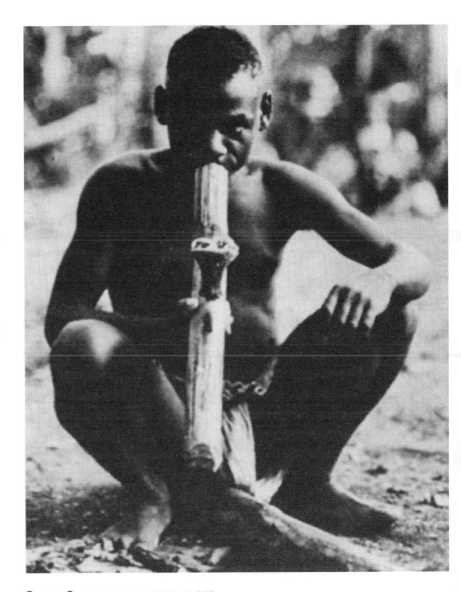

CONGO PYGMY WITH TRADITIONAL PIPE.

tion, rheumatic pains, female disorders, and absentmindedness. Those who understood its versatile medicinal properties probably also knew of its ability to elevate consciousness, although those secrets may have first been unlocked by

Chinese shamans and religious adepts. According to a book published by the cannabis-using Ethiopian Zion Coptic Church, a Taoist priest writing in the fifth century B.C. testified that cannabis was used by "necromancers, in combination with Ginseng, to set forward time and reveal future events." Also surviving are ancient warnings that hallucinations ("seeing devils") will plague those who overindulge in *Ma-fen,* or "hemp fruit," but that long-term usage helps "one communicate with spirits and lightens one's body."[3]

The oldest specific evidence of hemp consumption for spiritual purposes comes from India. Dating from roughly 1400 B.C.E. and containing far older material, the Indian religious text *Athharva Veda* mentions the sacred grass "bhang," the means by which one communes with Shiva, the deity of spiritual enlightenment in the Hindu trinity. The text implores the sacred plant to "deliver us from calamity" and to "protect . . . against diseases and all the Demons."[4] According to Indian tradition, the bhang plant was produced when the gods churned the heavenly ocean using Mount Mandara as a stirring stick. A drop of nectar spilled onto the earth, and hemp sprouted on the spot. Since the tenth century, this

bhang-nectar—a gift from the gods and a favorite of the gods Indra and Shiva—has been called Indracana. By 1300 B.C.E. recreational and religious use of hemp was common.

Cannabis use expanded from India into Persia and Assyria. As early as 900 B.C.E. the Assyrians used hemp for incense in an age when ceremonial herbs were burned for more than just their fragrance. The well-known religious scholar Mircea Eliade remarks that "shamanic ecstasy induced by hemp smoke was known in ancient Iran."[5] The continued use of incense in modern day rituals recalls a time when the psychoactive properties of incense were honored as a way to bring the worshipper in touch with supernatural forces.

The ancient Greeks and Romans generally preferred to intoxicate themselves with alcohol, but they traded with cannabis eaters and inhalers and knew of the plant's psychotropic effects. Writing in the fifth century B.C.E., the ancient Greek historian Herodotus observed that the Scythians threw hemp seed on heated stones in a closed tent as a postfuneral purification ritual. Herodotus noted, "The Scythians, transported with the vapor, shout aloud."[6] Perhaps Herodotus missed out on the shouting in his own land. His contemporary Democritus (ca. 460 B.C.E.) wrote that when the plant—known to him as *potamaugis*—was drunk with wine and myrrh it produced delirium, visionary states, and at times "immoderate laughter." Centuries later, about 200 C.E., the Roman physician Galen described the custom of sharing cannabis with guests to inject the occasion with joy and laughter.

Israelites living in the time of the Old Testament also transacted with the cannabis-using peoples that surrounded them, and although scholars seem divided as to whether or not cannabis is mentioned in the Old Testament, it takes no great stretch to believe that suggestions of its use are accurate. References to ritual incense abound, and the early Jews were no less likely than other early peoples to inhale herbal smoke for its psychoactive properties. Dr. C. Creighton, a British physician writing in 1903, maintains that the "honeycomb" in the Song of Solomon (5:1) and the "honey-wood" in 1 Samuel 14:25–45 are cannabis. In the latter reference, Jonathan dipped a rod in the honeycomb and "put his hand to his mouth and his eyes brightened."[7]

Widespread ritual use of hemp next shows up in the Middle East following the rise of Islam, which forbade the partaking of alcohol but made no mention of hemp and its derivatives. With no cultural prohibitions against its use, hashish consumption became commonplace. Its spiritual powers were prized particularly by the Sufis. According to one apocryphal story, a Sufi religious leader named Haider, who lived in the mountains of Rama around 500 C.E., accidentally discovered the plant's euphoric powers and shared them with his followers. His monk Sheraz told the disciples that God had bestowed upon them the "special favor" of a plant "which will dissipate the shadows which cloud your souls and brighten your spirits." As priest classes are wont to do, Haider asked his disciples to hide the plant's divine properties from the common folk. Whether beatific grins or loose lips betrayed the secret is not recorded. Nevertheless, Sufi poets were soon praising the virtues of "the cup of Haider" which had "the fragrance of amber and sparkles like a green emerald."[8]

Despite the lack of formal prohibitions, many Moslem priests preached to the masses about the evils of hashish, while in private indulging in their own secret stashes. In one old tale retold by Abel, a priest is in the midst of an animated sermon against the "vile drug" when his tunic falls open and a bag of the herb tumbles to the ground. Not missing a beat, the priest shouts to his startled audience, "This is the demon of which I have warned you; the force of my words have put it to flight. Take care that in leaving me, it does not throw itself on one of you and enslave you." When the holy man finishes his harangue, the crowd disperses; he picks up his bag, resecures it behind his tunic, and goes on his way.[9]

A funerary urn (detailed in chapter 4), believed to date from 500 B.C.E. and containing marijuana leaves and seeds, seems to be the earliest hard evidence of hemp use in Europe. The urn, suggests Abel, represents the influence of the Scythian cult of the dead on the Celts, whose culture dominated most of Europe at that time. But although hemp was highly prized for its medicinal properties, evidence of its use as a hallucinogen all but disappeared by medieval times. Most likely, however, it was simply forced underground by the expansion of Christianity. The ambitious Roman emperor Constantine converted to Christianity in the third century

and declared it to be the mandatory state religion, thereby adding the power of the early church to his own and extending the life of his crumbling empire. Fifty years later the emperor Theodosius the Great forbade the practice of all religions but Christianity, undoubtedly driving many hemp-consuming cults into the shadows. By the thirteenth century the Inquisition specifically outlawed hemp ingestion along with many other natural remedies; in the following century, the prohibitions spread to France. The use of cannabis—whether to commune with the divine or to heal or simply to celebrate—was branded witchcraft, for which practitioners could be severely punished, even put to death. Among those charged was Joan of Arc, whom the inquisitors accused of using several "witch" herbs, including cannabis, to hear voices.

In 1484 Pope Innocent VIII issued a papal fiat declaring hemp to be an unholy sacrament of "satanic masses" as part of the church's assault on Arabic culture in general. The ban, which lasted more than 150 years, did not go unchallenged. Benedictine monk and radical dissenter Francois Rabelais (1483–1553) satirized both church and state in the esoteric book series *Gargantua and*

Pantagruel (see chapter 4), in which "the herb Pantagruelion" is incontrovertibly hemp.

So stigmatized was the mind-altering use of hemp that it did not reemerge in Europe in any obvious manner until the mid-nineteenth century when its use assumed a less spiritual and more recreational focus. In 1845 French psychiatrist Dr. Jacques Joseph Moreau (de Tours) reported the results of experiments on hemp intoxication that he conducted by ingesting hashish, which he had brought back from Algeria. For the medical public, he described the experience—euphoria, hallucinations, flight of ideas, and incoherence—in sober clinical terms. To his friends, including the writer Theophile Gautier, he gushed, "Try *this!*" After following the doctor's advice, Gautier spread the good news to his bohemian circle of friends, including the Romantic writers Charles Baudelaire and Alexander Dumas. Before long the coterie was meeting regularly at the Hotel Pimodan as Le Club des Hachischins ("The Club of the Hashish Eaters") to munch *dawamesk,* a potent hashish candy, with their lavish dinners.

In an article written for *La Revue des Deux Mondes,* Gautier, clearly as intoxicated by his own literary powers as by the hashish itself, described one of his club evenings: "It seemed that my body had dissolved and become transparent. I saw inside me the hashish I had eaten in the form of an emerald which radiated millions of tiny sparks. All around me I heard the shattering and crumbling of multi-colored jewels. I still saw my comrades at times but as disfigured half plants half men."[9] Noting Gautier's overdramatic depiction of the events leading up to the meal, psychiatrist Lester Grinspoon, the author of several important books on psychoactive plants, commented: "There does not seem to be a great deal of difference between his descriptions of his perceptions while straight and those under the influence of the drug."[10]

The hashish reports of the troubled Baudelaire would seem to be less dependable even than Gautier's, although not without merit. He emphasizes, as would Timothy Leary and others a century later, the impact of both mind-set and physical setting on the hallucinogenic experience and distinguishes between the hashish hallucination, which "has its roots in the environment," and "true" hallucinations, which do not. But like his clubmate Gautier, Baudelaire also leaned toward hyperbole and other forms of liter-

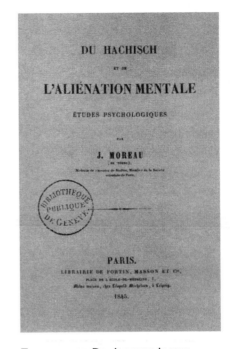

TITLE PAGE OF DR. JACQUES JOSEPH MOREAU'S *HASHISH AND MENTAL ILLNESS.*

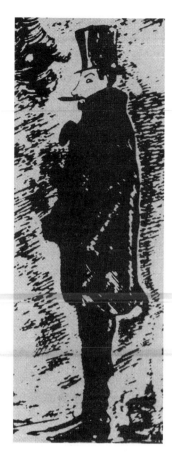

SELF-PORTRAIT OF CHARLES BAUDELAIRE, WHILE UNDER THE INFLUENCE OF HASHISH.

ary exaggeration. As Grinspoon and others have noted, his descriptions of an advanced hashish high sound more like a high dose of LSD or a meditator's merging with cosmic consciousness. In *Les Paradis artificiels* (1860), Baudelaire writes that the habitual hashish user "supposes himself to be the center of the Universe. . . . But soon this storm of pride changes to a calm, silent, restful beatitude; the universality of man is announced colorfully, and lighted as it were by a sulphurous dawn."[11]

Although hemp cultivation for industrial purposes dates back to 1629 in America, no clear record of its use as an intoxicant shows up until the mid-nineteenth century. Cannabis was widely used as a medicine by this time, and its ability to produce "exhilaration, intoxication, delirious hallucinations," and so on were catalogued in the United States *Dispensatory* in 1851. Five years later, a young American named Fitz Hugh Ludlow published an article in *Putnam's* magazine about his experiences as a hashish consumer. The next year, Harper Brothers published his tales, expanded into the book *The Hasheesh Eater*. Although Ludlow was undoubtedly a hashish user, scholars consider his writings even more fanciful than those of Gautier and Baudelaire, who probably influenced him.

In succeeding decades, underground bohemian hemp scenes appear to have flourished in many large American cities. The November 1883 edition of *Harper's New Monthly Magazine* featured an anonymous article titled "A Hashish-House in New York," in which the author describes a "house up-town where hemp is used in every conceivable form, and where the lights, sounds, odors, and surroundings are all arranged so as to intensify and enhance the effects." The writer—thought to be Dr. H. H. Kane, author of a medical text on morphine—reports that "smokers from different cities, Boston, Philadelphia, Chicago, and especially New Orleans, tell me that each city has its hemp retreat."[12]

In Baltimore cannabis was consumed even more openly. In a book published in 1894, Dr. George Wheelock Grover wrote of walking down a street in the leading business district and chancing upon a store sign advertising "Gungawalla Candy, Hashish Candy." He purchased a box and to test the potency took "a full dose." Three hours later, the effects surfaced while he was dining with medical friends and he reported his altered awareness to them, including his witnessing "hundreds of canary birds singing in gilded cages.[13]

Other reports of occasional recreational consumption continued until about 1920, when cannabis burst into wider use, following the implementation of Prohibition via the Eighteenth Amendment and the Volstead Act. In New York City, "tea pads" modeled after opium dens or speakeasies sprang up like weeds. Their congenial proprietors dispensed marijuana for as little as a quarter for customers who got high inside. In the South, New Orleans achieved wide notoriety as the port of entry and distribution center for cannabis from Havana, Tampico, and Vera Cruz. The onslaught of anti-marijuana legislation in the 1930s accomplished what anti-drug laws generally do—it expanded the market. Marijuana grew popular with jazz musicians, whose art was, like cannabis, a spiritual escape from the mundane. As they moved to northern cities from New Orleans, the jazzers carried their cannabis with them.

While marijuana use crept into the general public through such avenues as popular culture and the influence of cannabis-using musicians and artists, it also entered through more regimented company. During World War II and the Korean War, many soldiers became acquainted with the herb for the first time. Returning home after their tours of duty, many of them took advantage of the G.I. Bill to go to college, introducing cannabis to the fertile social enviroment on campuses all across America. Disgusted by the bland conformity of the suburban life to which their parents had consigned them, dismayed by the complacent values they observed in their parents' affluent lifestyles, middle-class American youth had begun to feel a tug at their souls. Something deep within them cried for a more authentic cultural destiny, one that was spiritual, not material in essence. Although this yearning wouldn't express itself as mass youth culture until a decade later, the pattern was established by the Beats of the 1950s, whose sacrament was marijuana. The Beats idealized the dreamy bohemian worlds of the past century and also the exotic urban cultures of jazz musicians and other artists, which seemed to offer attractive alternatives to the lives that their parents had mapped for them. In the 1960s, all of the cannabis-conducive dynamics birthed in previous decades—legal repression, alienation from prevailing social values, the appeal of bohemian and spiritual alternatives—joined with new and equally powerful social forces to spread cannabis use to nearly an entire generation. The policing efforts of governments, religious establishments, and threatened corporations notwithstanding, it appears that cannabis use for transcendent purposes will endure as an indelible feature of human existence.

"The Heavenly Guide": Hemp's Role in Spiritual Culture

In the Old World, remnants of the ancient, spiritually based hemp tradition survive alongside more contemporary forms of consumption. For example, in parts of Eastern Europe, the custom of tossing a handful of hemp seeds into a fire as an offering to the dead has survived its probable Scythian origin thousands of years before. In Poland and Lithuania, the custom persists of preparing a hemp-seed soup—called *semieniatka*—for the dead on Christmas Eve, when they are believed to visit their families. A striking number of cultures have made a connection between cannabis and reverence

for the dead, undoubtedly because of cannabis's seeming ability to transcend spatial and temporal boundaries.

Hemp use, which has touched nearly every major spiritual tradition on earth at some point in history, continues to play a prominent role in many traditions today. In several more obscure or esoteric traditions, its use is central. In contrast, most major religions of the West have disowned any mystical heritage in which cannabis use may have once played a part. As William Emboden notes in his book *Ritual Use of* Cannabis sativa *L.,* Western religious traditions tend to emphasize "sin, repentance, and mortification of the flesh." It is in older, non-Western religious cults where we find an unbroken custom of cannabis used as a euphoriant, "which allowed the participant a joyous path to the Ultimate; hence such appellations as 'heavenly guide.'"[14]

The following tracks the path of that heavenly guide through the world's major, and several minor, spiritual traditions.

HINDUISM

The Hindu scriptures among all spiritual literatures contain the oldest and most profuse direct references to cannabis as a divine intoxicant. As mentioned earlier, the Vedas identify bhang as the means by which one both communes with the god Shiva and frees oneself from sin. A scriptural story relates the myth of how Shiva and the cannabis plant came to be associated. After squabbling with his family, Shiva wanders into the fields to be alone. Oppressed by a fierce sun, he finds shade under a tall hemp plant and then crushes and eats some of its leaves. The snack so refreshes him that he adopts it as his favorite food, thereby becoming known as the "Lord of Bhang." According to J. M. Campbell, in an appendix to the *Indian Hemp Drugs Commission Report of 1893–1894,* "He who drinks bhang drinks Shiva. The soul in whom the spirit of bhang finds a home glides into an ocean of Being freed from the weary round of self-blinded matter."[15] He continued, "To the Hindu the hemp plant is holy. A guardian lives in the bhang leaf . . . To meet someone carrying bhang is a sure omen of success. To see in a dream the leaves, plant, or water of bhang is lucky; it brings the goddess of wealth into the dreamer's power . . . a longing for bhang foretells happiness." The seventeenth-century Hindu text, *Rajvallabha,* concurs that consuming this food of the

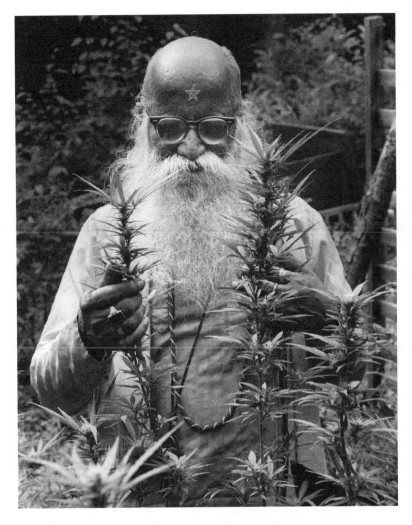

GANESH BABA, AN INDIAN SAINT, AT AGE 92, ADMIRING SOME OF THE SACRAMENTS OF HIS ORDER. PHOTOGRAPH BY IRA COHEN.

gods creates vital energy, increases mental powers, and brings delight to Shiva.

In ancient times the preparation of hemp resin was a secret of the Brahmin priests, who restricted its public use by allowing bhang to be used only occasionally and in limited quantities as an

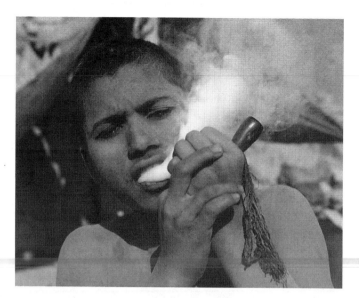

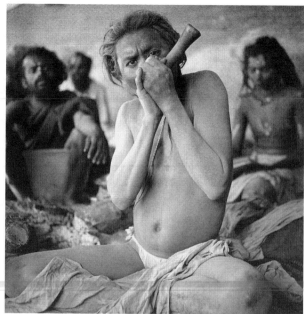

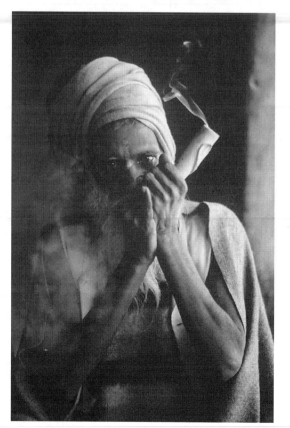

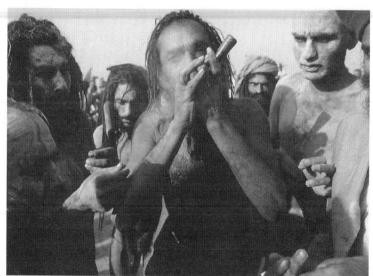

SADHUS WITH CHILLUMS. PHOTOGRAPHS BY KEVIN BUBRISKI.

offering in religious celebrations such as the Kali, Durja-Puja, and Vijaya Dasmi festivals. Among his myriad epithets, Shiva is known as Lord of Bhang, and on Shivram (Shiva's night) hot butter decoctions of bhang are poured over representations of the sacred Shiva Lingam all night long. On the final day of the Durja-Puja festival, the idols are thrown into the water, and the celebrants visit with friends and relatives. Hosts offer their visitors a cup of bhang drink and a dish of majoon sweets.

Historically, bhang became associated with Kali, a feminine aspect of Shiva, in medieval Tantric sex rituals. Campbell reported that worshipers of Vishnu—like Shiva, one of the Hindu trinity and a principal player in the Vedic myth about hemp's origin—often make offerings of bhang. The Sikhs, a Hindu offshoot dating back to 1500 that opposes the caste system and magic idolatry, also have a tradition of bhang consumption. Ernest Abel writes that bhang drinking was mandatory for Sikhs during the Dasehera holiday honoring the religion's founder.

Although disavowed by many Hindu spiritual leaders, particularly those who have established broad followings in the West, cannabis use continues among many Indian Hindus today in three forms: the bhang drink prepared from dried leaves; the sticky, potent flower tops called ganga; and the collected resins called charas, or hashish. In the *High Times Encyclopedia of Recreational Drug Use,* Michael Aldrich writes, "Most of India's wandering ascetics use cannabis constantly, drinking bowls of bhang to celebrate auspicious holidays and smoking fat chillums [pipes] of ganga at cremation pyres along the Ganges." Fulfilling a spiritual function described in the Vedas, the ascetics—called *sadhus*—radiate spiritual energy as they walk about the country, feeding the consciousness of India and the planet, and believe the use of bhang supplies them with spiritual power, brings them closer to enlightenment, and honors Shiva, who is said to be perpetually intoxicated by cannabis.

Voluntarily homeless, the sadhus live in the forest or in caves or walk perpetually, subsisting on alms. Their hair hangs in long matted strands, their skin is covered with dust or ashes, and they wear only a few rags or nothing at all. Sadhus practice physical austerities including celibacy and long fasts without food or water. Bhang is said to help them center their thoughts on the divine and to endure hardships. By reputation the sacred herb has

The Indian Hemp Trick

On numerous occasions over the centuries, including several times in recent decades, fakirs in India have allowed themselves to be buried alive without air, food, or drink before reliable, educated witnesses from the West. Days later, they are revived in front of those same witnesses, emerging from their internment in perfect health. Supposedly, no scientific explanation has ever fully accounted for the phenomenon, but perhaps overlooked in the rash of hypotheses is one first published in 1855, by the Bavarian scientist Baron Ernst von Bibra (1806–1878). In his book *Plant Intoxicants,* a detailed study of seventeen psychoactive plants, von Bibra suggests that hashish may be the fakir's secret:

Hibernating mammals prove indeed that a condition very similar to [a live burial] may occur in warmblooded individuals with an active metabolism. I was able to convince myself that such a condition can be artificially brought on or put off at will, by artificially changing the temperature. In man, however, such a condition can only be produced by narcotic means that cause his metabolism to slow down considerably. We noticed that, in all cases, small doses of hashish produce an increased appetite; large doses, on the other hand, may easily have the opposite results. It is possible that some of the fakirs possess a hemp preparation that enables them to undergo the described experiments.[16]

In support of von Bibra's idea, cannabis is reputed to help Hindu *sadhus* bear long fasts, and it also helps peasants to endure long periods of famine, as noted elsewhere.

helped the general population survive periods of famine as well.

Cannabis also fulfills other spiritual roles for the Hindu laity. On religious holidays—particularly those dedicated to Shiva—and at weddings, it aids Hindus of all classes in celebrating and consecrating the occasion. J. M. Campbell describes the common practice of students, yogis, and other religious practioners partaking of cannabis before contemplating the Mysteries. Not all sects advocate the use of bhang—or any other mind-altering substance, for that matter—but none condemn cannabis so long as it is not taken frivolously, devoid of religious intent.

BUDDHISM

In the Mahayana Buddhist tradition, legend has it that the Buddha lived on one cannabis seed a day in the six years of ascetic discipline prior to his enlightenment. But the involvement of cannabis in some types of Buddhist practice is more than just mythical, and it is contemporary as well as historical. For example, the Tantric Buddhists in the Tibetan Himalayas use cannabis ritually to deepen their meditation and raise awareness, according to Harvard botanical professor Richard Evans Schultes and LSD discoverer Albert Hofmann, two leading experts on psychoactive plants.

ISLAM

In his appendix to *The Indian Hemp Drugs Commission Report of 1893–1894,* J. M. Campbell made it clear that, to a large extent, what goes for Hindus and hemp also is true of Moslems:

> To forbid or even seriously to re-strict the use of so gracious an herb as hemp would cause widespread suffering and annoyance and to large bands of worshipped ascet-ics, deep-seated anger. It would rob the people of a solace in discom-fort, of a cure in sickness, of a guardian whose gracious protec-tion saves them from the attacks of evil influences, and whose mighty power makes the devotee of the Victorious, overcoming the demons of hunger and thirst, of panic, fear, of the glamour of Maya or matter, and of madness, able in rest to brood on the Eternal, till the Eternal, possessing him body and soul, frees him from the haunt-ing of self and receives him into the Ocean of Being. These beliefs the Musalman [Moslem] devotee shares to the full. Like his Hindu brother, the Musalman fakir reveres bhang as the lengthener of life, the freer from the bonds of self. Bhang brings union with the Di-vine Spirit. "We drank bhang and the mystery I am He grew plain. So grand a result, so tiny a sin."[17]

In the same appendix, Campbell described the practice of Trinath worship, common to both Hindus and Moslems, in which "the use of ganja is considered essential."

"It appears to be observed at all times," he continued,

> and at all seasons by Hindus and Muhammadans alike, the latter calling it Tinlakh Pir. . . . Originally one pice worth of betel nut was offered to the god. But now ganja—it may be in large quanti-ties—is preferred, and during the incantations and the performance of the ritual it is incumbent on all present to smoke.[18]

Still, Campbell asserts, the Mos-lem distinguishes between rever-ence for bhang and true worship, "which is due to Allah alone." In Is-lam, bhang represents not the spirit of the Almighty, but the spirit of the prophet Khizr, or Elijah.

The Sufis are the Moslems most associated with cannabis. In *Scan-dal: Essays on Islamic Heresy,* Peter Lamborn Wilson cites the Turkish Sufi poet Fuzuli, who claims that "hashish is the Sufi master him-self." Wilson notes that cannabis use has receded in modern Sufism, and has been banned en-tirely by some sects. But other modern day devotees still hold it in the original regard and use it in the original manner.

ZOROASTRIANISM

Zoroastrianism, which would profoundly influence Christianity, Islam, and later Judaism, dates to about 500 B.C.E. It arose in early Persia, but it derives from Hindu roots, even as it represents important departures from them. For example, as noted by authors Chris Bennett, Lynn Osburn, and Judy Osburn in *Green Gold, the Tree of Life: Marijuana in Magic and Religion,* "much of the *Zend-Avesta,* the book containing the teachings of . . . Zoroaster . . . comes directly from the Hindu Vedas."[19]

Considerable speculation exists that the substance *haoma,* central to Zoroastrian myth, is in fact hemp. The story of the birth of Zoroaster, the religion's mythical and perhaps historical founder, is drenched in haoma. The prophet's soul comes to earth with rain, which grows plants eaten by his parents' cows and transmutes his soul-body into milk. His parents drink a mixture of this milk and haoma, have intercourse, and conceive Zoroaster, who enters the world laughing.[20] Will Durant writes that Zoroaster, also known as Zarathustra, condemned the practice of haoma consumption that he encountered among his people in pre-Zoroastrian religious rituals. But Mircea Eliade suggests that Zoroaster was more likely upset not only by the bloody sacrifice of cows, which he considered sacred, but also by "orgiastic rites" and other excesses including immoderate haoma consumption attached to the ritual rather than haoma per se. Considering the role of the substance in the prophet's birth story, the conclusion makes sense.

When properly prepared and drunk in a pious manner, haoma is said to bestow wisdom, courage, success, health, long life, greatness, and protection from the ill will of others. Young women searching for husbands, married women hoping to conceive, and students seeking knowledge are advised to utilize its divining powers. Haoma is described as yellow or gold in color and growing on mountain slopes, traced by scholars to the Hindu Kush region. Bennett and colleagues point out that ripe hemp in the Middle East and India is of that same color and that the ganja of Hindu Kush is of legendary potency.[21]

At any rate, haoma references mysteriously fade away in the literature, to be replaced by direct celebration of bhang. In the *Zend-Avesta,* early Zoroastrian heroes Gustap and Ardu drink bhang in order to soul-travel to heaven and learn divine mysteries. The Magi of the Christian nativity story were

Zoroastrian adepts, so many hemp advocates speculate that cannabis may have been among the gifts brought to the infant Christ.

Today, Zoroastrianism survives mainly as the religion of the Gabars of Iran and Parsees of India. Hemp scholar Sula Benet notes that until recent times, Latvians and Ukrainians prepared a dish from hemp for "Three Kings Day." In the traditions of both cultures (and in Irish culture as well) can be found references to young women using hemp seed to predict their future husbands.

JUDAISM

As mentioned above, the ancient Jews surely transacted with cannabis-using cultures, and claims that their own religious practices remained free of psychoactive substances—besides sacramental wine—are suspect. Sula Benet writes that "the astonishing resemblance between the Semitic *kanbos* and the Scythian *cannabis* leads me to suppose that the Scythian word was of Semitic origin."[22] Other scholars have disputed the point, but etymologists at Hebrew University in Jerusalem concluded in 1980 that the Old Testament word *kineboisin* in fact meant cannabis. Embarrassed representatives of both the Jewish

and Christian mainstream pointed out that kineboisin was merely part of a holy anointing oil that God commanded Moses to apply externally (Genesis 30:23). But if cannabis use is acknowledged in this one instance, wouldn't it have been as obvious a choice for incense, which the Bible shows Jews using ritually up until about 300 B.C.E.?

AFRICAN TRADITIONS

Cannabis use, for both religious and more casual mind-altering purposes, abounds throughout the African continent. Although no one has been able to tie down a date of origin, the casual and ritual inhalation of cannabis smoke predates the arrival of Europeans. Known mainly as *dagga,* cannabis is a sacrament and medicine to the Pygmies, Zulus, and Hottentots. In ancient times, Ethiopia was known as the "Land of Incense"—this in a country still renowned for its potent hashish.

Ethiopian Christianity, in which cannabis use is common, predates even the formation of the Roman Catholic Church. But the Ethiopian Christian's use of cannabis in worship may go back farther still. The Ethiopian Zion Coptic Church maintains a cannabis-based Eucharist practice that its elders trace, through oral tradition, to their ancestors before the time of Christ.[23] When natives of this region were brought to Jamaica as slaves, they brought their cannabis spirituality with them, possibly sowing the seeds for its adoption by the modern day Rastafarian movement.

William Emboden, Jr., a prominent scholar of psychoactive plants, reports that the water pipe, used to cool and refine cannabis smoke, was developed in North Africa. Before the arrival of the Portuguese, Emboden writes, the people of the Zambezi Valley in the south of Africa would unite themselves as a community by inhaling the smoke of a smoldering pile of hemp.[24] Later, more advanced methods including water pipes upgraded this practice.

In the late nineteenth century, the Baloubas, a Bantu tribe that conquered much of the Belgian Congo, used dagga to unify the diverse subdued peoples into one. After first publicly destroying the traditional religious objects of the captured tribes, Chief Kalamba-Moukenge substituted dagga to promote harmony and cooperation between them. "So impressed were the formerly-warring factions," notes Emboden, "that they united under the name bena-Riamba—'sons of Cannabis.'"[25]

In contemporary North Africa,

many people maintain special rooms in their homes where kif is smoked while traditional stories, dances, and songs are passed to the young generation.

CHINESE TAOISM

Historian Joseph Needham attributes the establishment of Mount Shao, the first major center of Taoist practice (ca. 350 C.E.), in part to cannabis use by the sage Yang Hsi. Under the influence of the herb, Yang Hsi experienced a series of visions of Lady Wei, the Mao brothers, and other members of the pantheon who transmitted a number of sacred texts through him.[26] Unfortunately for hemp historians, the ancient Taoists wrote about the sacramental use of cannabis by others but not themselves. T'ao Hung-Ching, the most eminent Taoist magician of the fifth century noted in his book, Ming-i pieh-lu, that "the magicians say" if hemp seeds are consumed with ginseng it will endow one with the ability to see future events. Other Taoist texts document hemp use by magicians and alchemists as well.[27] For example, the sixth-century Taoist collection Wu Shang Pi Yao (Essentials of the Matchless Books) states that alchemists added hemp to their incense.

These texts along with other surviving resources indicate that Chinese shamans used cannabis widely for spiritual purposes during this time. A late edition of the Chinese materia medica *Pen Ts'ao,* attributed to the Emperor Shen Nung, asserts that if hemp is taken over a long period of time, one can communicate with the spirits. Adding to this prescription, the seventh-century physician Meng Shen advised that one must eat hemp seed for at least three months in order to see spirits in this way.[28]

Evidence of an exchange between Taoism and known hemp-using mystical traditions in Persia and India also exists, perhaps leading some scholars to speculate that the classic Taoist text *The Secret of the Golden Flower* contains numerous references to hemp. Consider the following advice about incense: "If there is time in the morning, one may sit during the burning of an incense stick, that is the best. In the afternoon, human affairs interfere and one can therefore easily fall into indolence."[29]

JAPANESE TRADITIONS

Sailors brought hemp to Japan, where it was called *asa* and played a role in many traditional rituals and stories. Shinto priests in an-cient Japan are said to have used ceremonial sticks—called *gohei*—with undyed hemp fibers attached to one end. Waving the fibers, which symbolized purity, above a person's head was thought to drive away any evil spirits residing inside him or her. Hemp also played a role in the marriage customs of earlier times. The groom's family would send hempen gifts to the bride's family to show she was acceptable to them. Strands of the fiber were arrayed at weddings as a symbol of a wife's obedience to her husband. Hemp advocate Jack Herer has found evidence of marijuana used in Shintoism to bind married couples together and grace their union with laughter and happiness. Advocate Chris Conrad's research indicates that Japanese Taoists used cannabis seeds in their incense burners by the first century C.E.

CHRISTIANITY

The puritanical orientation of modern day Christianity against psychotropics may well betray the bent of its earliest history. In particular, the Christian tradition of the Eucharist may derive from earlier sacramental traditions—in Hinduism, Zoroastrianism, and so on—in which hemp and other psychoactive substances were employed. Some commentators suggest, with decent logic if not much hard evidence, that Jesus may have learned the ceremony directly from other hemp-using sects—perhaps the Gnostics, although their own knowledge about hemp is also inferred, not documented. The same train of logic might lead one to guess that the early Eucharist ceremonies might have included hemp itself.

WESTERN OCCULTISM, HERMETICISM, AND MYSTICISM

Because of aggressive policing and repression by a disapproving Church, explicit mentions of cannabis in Europe are rare from the Middle Ages through the mid-nineteenth century. However, early occultists and alchemists likely knew about, and advantaged themselves, of cannabis's spiritual attributes, as many of their spiritual descendants clearly did. In *Green Gold, the Tree of Life* the authors suggest that both the early Rosicrucians and Freemasons learned of the powers of cannabis through their contact with Arab sources. Medieval esoteric and alchemical texts contain profuse references to Sufism and Zoroastrianism, two traditions tied intimately to psychoactive plants including cannabis. And, of course, the writings of Francois Rabelais brought to the surface the formerly covert association of cannabis with esoteric knowledge.

Among later occultists, Aleister Crowley (1875–1947) wrote rapturously about cannabis in his 1907 essay, "The Psychology of Hashish," stating that the act of "exalting myself mystically and continuing my invocations while the drug dissolved the matrix of my diamond Soul" constituted "the supreme ritual of all religions." Among his students and hashish initiates was science fiction writer H. G. Wells. The poet W. B. Yeats also frequented esoteric circles, where he encountered Crowley and fellow occultists Dion Fortune and A. E. Waite. Yeats describes his hashish experiences in "The Trembling of the Veil" (1926). The Russian mystic George Gurdjieff (1877–1949), who obtained much of his knowledge of transcendent methodology from Sufi and other dervish sources, wrote openly about hashish in *Meetings with Remarkable Men* and is said to have used it with students to introduce them to the experience of awakening consciousness.

RASTAFARIAN MOVEMENT

Founded in the 1930s, the Jamaica-based Rastafarian movement is the most obvious example of cannabis employed for holy purposes. Vitally spiritual but more than a religion, Rastafarianism also functions as a social, cultural, and political philosophy for its followers, and ganga smoking lies at its core. Rastas—adherents of Rastafarianism—claim that ganga is the "healing of the nation" and "wisdom weed," finding scriptural justification for their view in the Western bible, much as do the Egyptian and Ethiopian Coptics.[30] They believe that smoking cannabis in a ritual manner cleanses both body and mind, preparing the user for meditation, prayer, the reception of wisdom, reasoning, and communal harmony with others, a central value for Rastas.

Rastafarianism, which celebrates the black Jamaican's African heritage, has its roots in a fascination with Ethiopia, itself a center of cannabis-influenced religious culture represented by the Ethiopian Coptic tradition. The teachings of Marcus Garvey, who pointed to Ethiopia as a symbol of freedom, sovereignty, and African spirituality, paved the way for Rastafarianism. Indeed, Rastas believe that the late Ethiopian emperor Haile Selassie was God reincarnated, fulfilling Garvey's prophesy that the crowning of a black king in Africa would identify the Redeemer.

But Rastafarian ties to Ethiopia and ganga spirituality may run deeper still. Some Jamaican Coptic elders claim that their beliefs first traveled to Jamaica when their ancestors were brought over in the 1800s as slaves. Hindu influence, via migrant workers from India, cannot be ruled out either. When black slaves gained their freedom in the British Caribbean in the mid-nineteenth century, indentured laborers from India came over to replace them. There they found hemp growing wild, the result of an abandoned industrial hemp project started by the British in 1800. Among the many Rasta words for cannabis—herb, iley, I-Shence, Kaya, lambsbread, and so on—are two distinctly Hindu-sounding names: ganga and Kali.

Cannabis and Mystical Sexuality

Throughout its long history of human use, cannabis has been associated with sexuality, both for pure sensual enjoyment and in the mystical, Tantric sense of sancti-

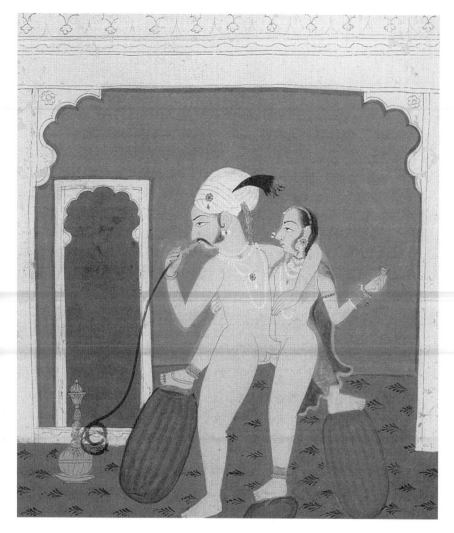

A NINETEENTH-CENTURY ILLUSTRATION OF THE USE OF CANNABIS IN TANTRA.

either reduces their interest in sex or just puts them to sleep! According to the holistically oriented medical writer Andrew Weil, "The experiences of people who smoke marihuana are astounding in their variety because marihuana has such slight intrinsic activity compared to other substances and is neither a pronounced sedative nor a stimulant." Cannabis's "unimpressive pharmacology," writes Weil, makes atmosphere especially crucial to users' experience.[31] Weil believes that cannabis is clearly *not* an aphrodisiac, a conclusion that virtually every researcher who has examined the matter has also reached. By the same token, cannabis can raise the sexual experience of the sensually inclined to divine proportions. Cannabis-loving lovers find that the herb amplifies sexual sensations, delays ejaculation in men, and enhances the sense of two being joined as one. No wonder then that cannabis and Tantra themselves became joined.

Adherents of Tantra, a Pan-Indian movement of the second century that influenced both Hinduism and Buddhism, uses sexuality as a means of ascending to the superconscious state. Mircea Eliade explains that the original philosophers of Tantra felt that the spirit was so "thickly veiled by the flesh,"

fied physical union. Its reputation in the first instance helps explain its use in the latter.

The ability of cannabis to stimulate and enhance sexual experience has been much heralded in some quarters, derided in others: some consider cannabis to be an aphrodisiac, while others claim it

in what was for them modern times, that the seeker "must therefore 'go back to the source' and, to that end, start from the fundamental, specific experiences of his blighted condition—in other words, the very sources of his life."[32] But not just any sex would do. Tantric intercourse must be meditative and focused on an experience of oneness, not orgasm. For those purposes, cannabis must have appeared to the original Tantrists a nearly indispensable aid.

As described by Ernest Abel, the cannabis prelude to yogic sex would begin ninety minutes before intercourse. With a bowl of bhang before them, the devotees would chant the mantra *Om hrim*—which invokes the image of the goddess Kali, to whom the sex is consecrated—and plead for occult power, or *siddhi.* Following several more mantras, the seekers would drink the mixture and engage in ritual love making.

The Sufis and Gnostic Christians are also known to have spawned—in opposition to their ascetic traditions—sects that practiced spiritualized sexuality, with Indian Tantric ideas a likely influence. For example, according to Barbara Walker in *The Woman's Encyclopedia of Myths and Secrets,* the Gnostic Great Mother Sophia is to Christ as Kali is to the Hindu Shiva,

the feminine aspect of an androgynous divinity. The two religions share similar ideas of enlightenment as well, says Walker, the Gnostic *apolytrosis,* or release, corresponding to the Hindu *moksha,* or liberation. Given the Sufis' known taste for cannabis and the Gnostics' suspected use, plus the anti-ascetic bent of mystic sex in general, cannabis can reasonably be supposed to have played a part in these practices too.

Child of the Goddess: Hemp and the Worship of the Great Mother

From the perspective of mystic spirituality, the history of human religion is regressive, not progressive. Religious history—as represented by the rise of modern Christianity and Judaism—moves away from a harmony with nature and away from personal enlightenment and the means for attaining it. What gets lost in the process is appreciation for the powers of the feminine, represented in ancient religions as the Great Mother or Goddess principle. And it is no coincidence that

And You Thought It Was the Broomstick?

Some sources suggest that cannabis, along with a slew of other psychotropic plants, contributed to the folk legend about flying witches, from which the Halloween image of witches on broomsticks stems. The following is a recipe for an ointment that these researchers say may have been applied intravaginally—with, yes, a broomstick—during witches' sabbaths:

TRADITIONAL ENGLISH FLYING OINTMENT

3 grams annamthol
30 grams betel
50 grams extract of opium
15 grams of cinquefoil
15 grams henbane
15 grams belladonna
15 grams hemlock
5 grams cantharidin
250 grams *Cannabis indica*

Blend with oil of your choice or butter.[33]

Cantharidin, by the way, is Spanish Fly, not at all out of place at these notoriously orgiastic affairs. If not actual flying, this formula might well have produced a rather erotic brand of astral traveling.

95

when religions begin repressing women, in heaven and on earth, they also begin to prohibit the use of psychotropic plants for religious purposes.

The ancients celebrated the Feminine. They recognized the image of the Mother in the earth that brought forth life and sustenance. The earth also birthed a special class of plants that nourished the spirit as well as the body and opened the gates to the great mysteries of creation. These too the ancients associated with the Feminine, or at least with androgyny. We can see these relationships most clearly in Hinduism, in which cannabis is identified with both Shiva and his female consort, who are often depicted in sexual union. At other times, Shiva is shown as androgynous, having a male build with female breasts and facial features.

Later, Buddhism and Gnostic Christianity were among the religions that adopted these concepts, and also—at least in the case of Buddhism, and probably in that of the Gnostics as well— the use of psychotropics like cannabis. But the Gnostics were driven underground in the Middle Ages when the organized Roman Catholic church banned Goddess worship and psychotropic rituals such as incense burning. From the

mystic's standpoint, the darkness hasn't yet lifted.

More compellingly than any other writer, Terence McKenna draws on these ancient themes to construct his vision of a more harmonious future:

Our present global crisis is more profound than any previous historical crises, hence our solution must be equally drastic. I propose that we should adopt the plant as the organizational model for life in the twenty-first century, just as the computer seems to be the dominant mental/social model of the late twentieth century, and the steam engine was the guiding image of the nineteenth century.

This means going back in time to models that were successful 15,000 to 20,000 years ago. When this is done it becomes possible to see plants as food, shelter, clothing, and sources of education and religion.[34]

McKenna names his vision the Archaic Revival, which incorporates

the rebirth of the Goddess and the ending of profane history . . . agendas that implicitly contain within themselves the notion of our re-involvement with and the emergence of the vegetable mind.

. . . Returning to the bosom of the planetary partnership means trading the point of view of the history-created ego for a more maternal and intuitional style.[35]

Such reinvolvement is, of course, to be guided by the teacher-gurus of the plant kingdom, the psychotropics.

The Secular Perspective

In addition to promoting mystic spirituality, cannabis has played a prominent role, particularly in recent history, in raising consciousness in a more worldly sense. The same quality of cannabis—of creating the ability to see everything in a novel way—that can produce almost incapacitating hilarity also opens the eyes and minds of some users to new, more serious possibilities culturally, politically, aesthetically, and intellectually. Suddenly, all previous assumptions are up for grabs and the chance juxtapositions and absurdities of the world become the stuff of completely unbounded mind-play. The conclusions reached—or the songs composed, or the poems written—under the influence of cannabis don't always hold up the next day, but when they do, they can be profound.

This is not to say that expansion of consciousness is automatic or intrinsic with marijuana or hashish. Andrew Weil points out that in the nineteenth century doctors in England and America commonly handed out tinctures of cannabis to patients for a variety of complaints. Not only did the practice not contribute to mass consciousness-raising, but few patients even reported getting intoxicated, "probably because they did not expect to and so ignored the psychoactive effects."[36] Cannabis, like more powerful hallucinogens, tends to amplify qualities that were already present in the user. For those who feel stuck in a rut of bland convention and wish to break free, cannabis has the power to grant their wish. For those with minds already opened a crack, the crack widens under the influence of cannabis. In historical circumstances where cannabis has made a big difference in social terms, it may have been planted in already fertile ground.

A brief review of the spiritual history of cannabis demonstrates this reciprocal relationship between cannabis and personal and social change. Historically, those who have most loudly proclaimed the mind-altering powers of cannabis have been cultural outsiders

Hemp Scholarship—The Case for Passionate Prejudice

Speculation and assumption necessarily rule most early histories of cannabis as a heavenly guide. Its first uses would, of course, have gone unrecorded. For thousands of years following, the surviving historical record is spotty and vague.

How then do we interpret? Most cannabis historians come from the ranks of either academic religious studies or the sciences such as botany or psychiatry. Following their rigid academic training, they only presume cannabis use where the record is explicit or where the identity of the plant can be safely inferred. With a few notable exceptions, they don't, for example, find cannabis references sprinkled throughout the Old and New Testaments the way some less conservative commentators, mainly passionate hemp advocates, do.

However, it's not impossible to justify the advocates' more freely associating approach. In general, the fervor common to defenders of the faith tends to cloud their judgment, particularly in the matter of interpreting ambiguous information. But in the case of cannabis research, the more dispassionate scholars may well be infected with a bias of their own. In their book *Green Gold, the Tree of Life: Marijuana in Magic and Religion,* authors and hemp advocates Chris Bennett and Lynn and Judy Osburn cite the relevant view of philosophy professor Stanley Moore. Consulted during a 1993 court case involving cannabis-smoking members of the Israel Zion Coptic Church, Moore suggested that the Coptics' claims about cannabis use in the Bible may indeed be accurate: "Western Jews and Christians, who shun psychoactive drugs in their faith practices, are the exception, not the norm."[37]

and elites—shamans, priests, religious devotees, artists, writers, bohemians, and musicians. Such people start off seeing, or at least desiring to see, things differently than the masses. Cannabis adds velocity to a process already well under way. In the West, the names Rabelais, Crowley, Baudelaire, Gautier, Rimbaud, Yeats, Ginsberg, and Kerouac—dedicated social dissenters all—stand out. The ganga-smoking Rastas of Jamaica are dedicated political and cultural rebels who shun even the term "Rastafarianism" because it smacks of organized, conventional religion. For the Beats, marijuana was more than just a window into Eastern mysticism or a bond with the idolized jazz musician or African-American; it was a protest against all that was wrong with the bourgeois world, and their heightened perceptions while intoxicated only turned up the volume on what they heard and felt when straight.

The most profound example of the ability of marijuana to raise mass social consciousness occurred during the Vietnam War era, on both the home front and the battle front. The spread of marijuana use to almost an entire generation of middle-class youth who came of age in the 1960s is inextricable from the dramatic changes in social, political, spiritual, and cultural values that mark that era. Cannabis did not kidnap them or their collective consciousness: the generation was ready for marijuana. It was almost as if the gods Shiva and Dionysus had descended in the form of the female plant cannabis. These long-haired gods of intoxication and ecstasy are known in the East and West for their frenzied dancing, rejection of city life, and support of animals and the natural world. Representing the wild and free nature of humanity, they are also the gods that break down the conventions and barriers of society.

The following are just some of the ways that cannabis, with other psychedelic drugs, contributed to convulsive change in the 1960s:

- As they had for the Beats in the 1950s, the spiritual properties and heritage of cannabis interested youth in a variety of alternatives to the rejected religions of their parents: classical mysticism like Hinduism, Taoism, and Native American spirituality, or occult esoterica like astrology and Tarot—to name just a few.
- The communal rituals of smoking cannabis, as well as the shared communal-utopian consciousness that the experience helped inspire, led to the formation of many spiritually based experiments in communal living, some of which endured such as The Farm in Tennessee.
- When young people raised in the suburbs wandered joint-in-mouth into nature, many noticed things about mountains and rivers and trees that they had completely missed on childhood trips with their parents or the scoutmaster. This new appreciation for the sublime beauty and intelligence of the natural world gave birth to numerous cultural forms, including interest in natural health, sustainable agriculture, renewable energy sources, organic dwelling concepts, antinuclear protest, and ultimately comprehensive environmentalism. You certainly can't attribute the entire environmental movement to expanded awareness on hemp, but it's safe to say that it was the influence of natural psychedelics like cannabis that first sensitized many nascent environmentalists to the fragile interdependence and irreplaceable grandeur of nature.
- Intellectuals who smoked cannabis, which encourages relativistic, fluid thought associations, discovered the wonders of whole-systems thinkers like Buckminster Fuller and Gregory Bateson and genre-busting theorists like Marshall McLuhan and Claude Lévi-Strauss.
- The peace movement greatly expanded its following thanks

to a plant that furthered peaceful, communal, sensitive behavior. The movement for more community-oriented, progressive approaches to capitalism is largely a product of the cannabis-using baby boom generation.

Many of these trends have, along with their trendsetters, matured into permanent features of the cultural landscape. The middle-class countercultural rebels of the 1960s are now middle-aged, but many hold onto their dreams of contributing to the creation of a more cooperative society, and many of those dreams have become manifest. The mass interest in holistic health; the profusion of socially considerate businesses; the development of resource-conserving, sustainable technologies, (some of them originally invented and tested by crafty backwoods hemp farmers); the expansion of progressive educational alternatives and secular homeschooling; the growth of vigorous nonprofit organizations with roots in 1960s and 1970s battles for environmentalism, peace, and social justice; the continuing interest of millions in mystical religion and personal growth; experiments with communal housing alternatives; the continued expansion of organic agricultural methods and markets; and the current re-awakening of interest in the industrial and medical utility of hemp itself—all of these social developments owe much to the cannabis-smoking counterculture that arose nearly three decades past.

The Pros and Cons of Hemp-Based Spirituality

Any discussion of the advantages and disadvantages of cannabis consumption must begin by re-asserting the essential harmlessness of the substance from a physical and psychological standpoint. A standard psychiatric reference states that cannabis produces neither physical dependence, withdrawal symptoms, a strong psychological dependence, nor a need by the user to increase the dose as he or she grows used to the drug.[38] Nearly every study undertaken of cannabis has shown it to be the most benign intoxicant in common usage. The few studies that have reached opposite conclusions have been suspect in methodology—not to mention motivation—and have not been replicated, costing them the respect of the wider scientific community.

The decision about whether to

use cannabis for spiritual or consciousness-raising purposes is far more ambiguous. Obviously, many spiritual leaders entirely reject the appropriateness of cannabis for spiritual practice; on the other hand, vast numbers of people have found their spiritual commitment and curiosity deepened after first using marijuana.

The standard advice given by spiritual leaders who are open to cannabis and other psychedelics is that while these substances may introduce some seekers to the possibilities of higher consciousness they can't deliver enlightenment itself. In *The Master Game,* Robert De Ropp offers his own version of this moderate point of view:

> It is *physiologically* lawful to obtain information about the workings of one's own organism by any means that does not damage the organism or render its possessor a slave to the procedure in question (physically dependent on a drug, for example). It is *psychologically* (or spiritually) lawful to obtain such information as part of a life game, the aim of which is realization of higher states of awareness. It is not spiritually lawful to take psychedelics merely for "kicks" or to use them as substitutes for the kind of inner work that alone can produce lasting results. Those who use the drugs in this way . . . commit [themselves] to a descending spiral. . . . Finally, the power to reascend is lost altogether.[39]

In some circles, however, the suspicion has long existed that the great sages do in fact know how to access the highest states with drugs but keep the secret to themselves to protect the information from misuse by the masses. Indeed, mystical traditions do typically maintain an inner, secret set of practices not intended for mass consumption but available to advanced students sometimes by intuition alone. Read the mystical literature carefully and the plot thickens. For example, a student of the Russian mystic Gurdjieff wrote that his Master alluded to a "pill" that could accomplish what might take an ascetic a month of austerities. No mystic disputes that the ultimate spiritual goal is to realize a capacity for cosmic consciousness that is entirely inside the seeker and that the seeker has the ability to reach that state entirely with his or her own inner resources. But will a second, labor-saving key, harvested from outside one's person, unlock that same door? That remains the intriguing question.

4

A GLOBAL
HISTORY
OF HEMP

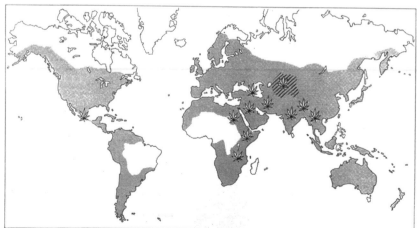

HEMP'S ORIGINAL HOME (HATCHED) AND AREAS IN WHICH IT NOW THRIVES (SHADED).

The history of mankind does not exist in a vacuum. Our story is interwoven with the stories of countless other species, and as we make these wild plants and animals a part of our lives, both our course and theirs change forever. If we are to understand our future, then, we must look to many pasts. By understanding these other stories, we help to explain our own.

No plant has had as complex a relationship with humanity as has hemp. Hemp's remarkable story does more than develop docilely beside our own; instead it weaves back and forth across our trail, disappearing entirely at times, only to reappear when least expected, often from an entirely new angle. It begins, appropriately, back at the beginning.

China

Hemp probably evolved in central Asia, where it became the first fiber plant to be cultivated. Cotton from India and Mediterranean flax were not introduced until thousands of years later. At this nascent stage of civilization, hemp was one of the threads that held communities together. Humans had previously tamed crops (including hemp) for food, but hemp gave them material readily available for the crafts they had begun to master. The masses relied on hemp for all their clothing; only the wealthy could afford the luxury of silk. Hemp and mulberry (the food of silkworms) were such important and widespread crops that the phrase "land of mulberry and hemp" was synonymous with China.

An abundance of evidence from burial pits and other sites throughout China demonstrates the continuous cultivation of Asian hemp from prehistoric times. A twelve-thousand-year-old Neolithic site unearthed at Yuan-shan (in what is now Taiwan) included remains of coarse, sandy pottery with hempen cord marks covering the surface, along with an incised, rod-shaped stone beater used to pound hemp. A late Neolithic site (circa 4000 B.C.E.) in Zhejiang

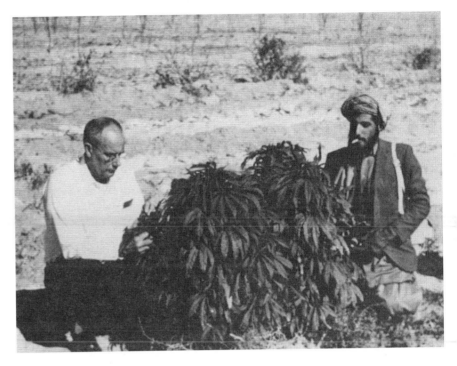

WILD HEMP NEAR KANDAHAR, AFGHANISTAN. PHOTOGRAPH BY R. E. SCHULTES.

province provides evidence of several textile articles made of hemp and silk. Remnants of a hemp-weaving industry emerged from excavation of a site of the Shang culture (1400–1100 B.C.E.) at Taixi Village in Hebei province, which produced a few fragments of burnt hemp fabric and a roll of hemp cloth in thirteen pieces.[1]

More than a thousand mortuary objects were recovered from a Chou tomb site at Hsin-Ts'un, near An-Yang. The inventory listed articles of hemp among those of gold, jade, marble, silk, lacquer,

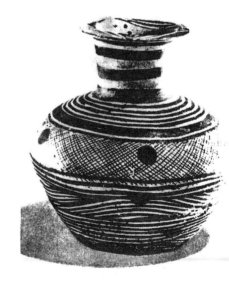

ANCIENT POTTERY WITH HEMPEN CORD MARKS, CHINA.

and other valuable materials. The inner coffin was made of wooden planks reinforced with bands of hemp cloth, which were fastened to the coffin with lacquer. A late Western Chou dynasty grave discovered in Shaanxi province contained bronze vessels, weapons, jade, pottery, and a tightly woven fragment of hemp cloth. At other Chou cemetary sites, bronze objects were found protected with silk and hemp textile wrappings.[2]

Sometimes ancient books make the best archaeologists. Several offer a glimpse at the role of hemp in early China. The *Shu Ching* (circa 2300 B.C.E.) states that the land in Shantung province is "whitish and rich . . . with silk, hemp, lead, pine trees, and strange stones . . ." and that in the Henan Valley people paid tribute to their rulers with hemp. The warlords' armies were dressed in armor sewn with hemp cord, and hemp bowstrings were so superior to the bamboo strings they replaced that they decided many a battle. Hemp was grown around every lord's castle to secure his military strength.[3]

The oldest pharmacopoeia in existence, the *Pen-Ts'ao Ching*, was compiled in the first or second century B.C.E. from more ancient fragments attributed to the legendary Emperor Shen Nung (circa 2300 B.C.E.), and that book mentions that hemp "grows along rivers and valleys at T'ai-shan, but it is now common everywhere."[4]

The *Shih Ching* (Book of Odes), a compilation of 305 songs and psalms composed between 1000 and 500 B.C.E., mentions millet thirteen times, mulberry twenty times, and hemp seven times. In the first dictionary, *Shuo-wen chieh-tzu,* compiled by Hsu Shen in the Eastern Han period, four variations for *ma* (hemp) are given. The *Chi-chiu-pien,* a primer composed in the first century B.C.E. for teaching reading and writing, lists rice, millet, and hemp in one sentence.[5]

These early books were limited by the bulk and weight of wooden and bamboo tablets and the expense of the rare silken "protopaper" *zhi.* During the Han Dynasty (207 B.C.E.–220 C.E.) it was discovered that the fibers of hemp made an inexpensive and nearly weightless writing surface when pounded together with mulberry bark. The dynastic history *Hou-Han Shu* attributes the invention of paper in 105 C.E. to Marquis Cai Lun, Prefect of the Masters of Techniques during the reign of Emperor He Di. Archaeologists have recovered older specimens of hemp paper from the Western and Eastern Han periods in Xinjiang, Inner Mongolia, and Shaanxi, however, so it is apparent that Cai Lun only supervised the art of papermaking by craftsmen, though he also worked to promote its use in the imperial bureaucracy. According to chapter 108 of the *Hou-Han Shu,* "He submitted the process to the emperor in the first year of Yuan-Hsing and received praise for his ability. From this time, paper has been in use everywhere."[6]

Several archaeological finds support the literary evidence of the *Hou-Han Shu.* The excavation of a ruined watchtower in Tsakhortei unearthed a specimen of paper bearing writing contemporary with Cai Lun. Other remarkable specimens were discovered in a tomb in Kansu province in 1974. The excavated pieces of hemp paper were found nailed in three layers with wooden strips on the sides of an oxcart. Perhaps the oldest specimens of paper extant, dating more than a century earlier than Cai Lun, were discovered in a tomb near Xian in Shaanxi province. The date of the tomb and the objects is no later than the reign of Wu Di of the Western Han Dynasty (140–87 B.C.E.). A fragment of the *Lun Yu* (Analects) of Confucius, written in 716 C.E. on bleached white hemp paper, was found in a cemetery at

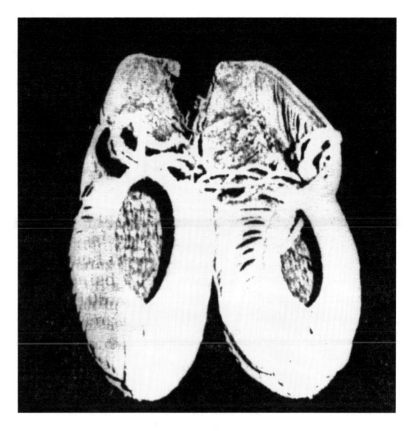

HEMP SHOES FROM A GRAVE IN TIRFAN, CHINA, 716 C.E.

Tirfan in Sinkiang province. The same site also yielded a beautiful pair of hemp paper shoes sewn with hemp threads. In 770 hemp was there again to help mankind make its next step—the printing of the first book, *Dharani,* a collection of prayers, on paper composed entirely of hemp.

Hemp paper is pliable, tough, fine, and waterproof and these characteristics made it popular and preferred for use in official documents, books, and calligraphy. The *Hsin*

Thang Shu says that the Chin Dynasty court provided the scholars in the Academy of Assembled Worthies with five thousand sheets of hemp paper each month. Hemp paper made in I-Chou (modern Szechuan) was used for all the books in the imperial library in the Khai-Yuan period (713–742 C.E.).

A few fragments of early Korean hemp paper have been recovered by archaeologists, including a thick, strong, bleached and glossy piece of *chi-lin chih* (paper from the Silla kingdom). This was an item of tribute to the Chinese, whose scholars and artists prized its fine quality. The *Fei Fu Yu Lueh* notes that Ming artist Tung Chi-Chang used *chi-lin chih* for his paintings.

Hemp is given extensive treatment in the *Fan Sheng-chih shu,* a treatise on farming written by Fan Sheng-chih about 25 B.C.E. The seeds of hemp were pretreated by immersing them in a decoction of powdered horse bones, aconite, silkworms, and sheep dung.[7] Although the Southern Ch'i (470–502 C.E.) dynastic history *Nan-Ch'i shu* mentions a porridge made of hemp seed, the use of hemp seed as a food staple diminished greatly by the sixth century. Eventually it was replaced by less oily grains, and its nutritional value was largely forgotten. Chinese farmers also used hemp seed to produce a black dye for their clothes.

Hemp also figures in the history of Chinese medicine. The great physician Hua Tuo (141–208 C.E.) formulated *ma-yo* (hemp wine) and *ma-fei-san* (hemp boiling powder), made with cannabis and aconite, for use as an anesthetic during the surgeries he performed.[8]

The materia medica *Pen Ts'ao* classifies *ma* as both yin (female, *chu-ma*) and yang (male, *i-ma*). Emperor Shen Nung classified *chu-ma* as one of the Superior Elixirs of Immortality, and he advised the Chinese to cultivate only the female plant because of its greater medicinal virtue. Court etiquette during the Zhou Dynasty (770–221 B.C.E.) required visitors to include *ma fen* among the ceremonial gifts. During the Qi Dynasty (479–502 C.E.), the roguing of the flowering male plants from hemp crops was a spectacular public ritual.

The peerless fiber of hemp is at the very core and epitome of Chinese culture—in the making of lacquerware. Chinese lacquer is made from the sap of a tree *(Rhus verniciferas)* which is strained through a sheet of hempen cloth to purify it. Then it is heated and stirred to homogenize and thicken it for application over a core of hemp fiber. Excavation of an Early Western Han tomb at Lao-fu-shan in Kiansi province uncovered more than two hundred grave goods including seventy lacquered items, among which were several winged cups on hemp-cloth cores.[9]

In the ninth century, female ambassadors from the "Country of Barbarians" (Indochina) presented the emperor with tribute, which they asserted "was made from refined water fragrant hemp." The court described it as "shining and radiant, infecting men with its sweet-smelling aroma. With this, and the intermingling of the Five Colors in it, it was more ravishingly beautiful than the brocades of our Central States."[10]

India and the Middle East

The Chinese may have been the first people to make use of hemp's fiber, but it was in India that the more lofty qualities of the plant were first fully appreciated. As we saw in the previous chapter, hemp became such an integral part of the Hindu religion that bhang and Shiva became inseparable. Indian mythology says that hemp was present with Shiva at the begin-

ning of the world, and, since modern science believes the plant may have originated somewhere around the Himalayas, we have no reason to doubt this.

Even in India hemp was not always used in a religious setting. Warriors were known to drink bhang to calm their nerves before battle, and, as everywhere else the plant was cultivated, hemp was used to cure a wide range of ills.

The earliest known Aryan name for hemp is *bhanga*, derived from the Aryan word *an* or *bhanj* meaning "to break." The modern term *cannabis* developed from the Sanskrit *sana* or *cana*. The regional name Bengal means "bhang land," and Bangladesh means "bhang land people."[11]

The Aryans who invaded India also penetrated the Middle East and spread into Europe as far west as France, sowing hemp seed wherever they went. But hemp had beaten them to Mesopotamia. One of the oldest archaeological relics in existence is a fragment of hemp cloth found at Çatal Hüyük that dates to about 8000 B.C.E. The plant is mentioned in Assyrian texts, where it is called *qu-nu-bu*, a "drug for grief." Other formulas used *qu-nu-bu* as a stomachic, aphrodisiac, poultice for swelling, and as a fumigant. The Phrygian tribes who

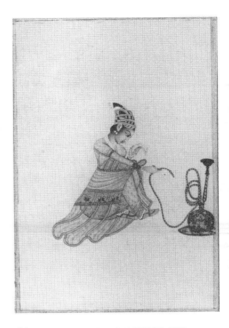

NOBLEMAN SMOKING A WATER PIPE. 18TH CENTURY, INDIA.

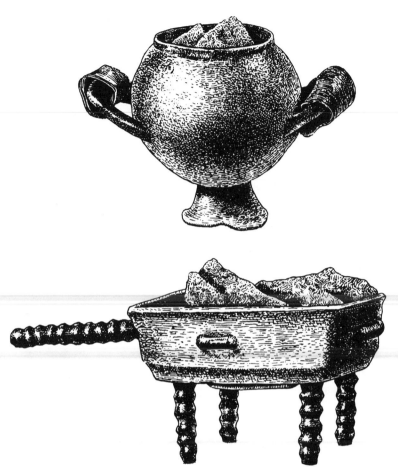

POT CONTAINING HEMP (TOP) AND CENSER FOR BURNING HEMP, FROM SCYTHIAN GRAVE SITE.

in the library of the Babylonian emperor Ashurbanipal. *Qu-nu-bu* is mentioned in a letter (preserved in the royal archives) written to the mother of Assyrian King Esarhaddon about 680 B.C.E. In Persia the seeds of hemp were called *shahdanah*, or "emperor's seeds."[12]

The westward spread of hemp's popularity was greatly helped by the Scythians, an offshoot of the Aryans who invaded India. The Scythians swept from Siberia into the middle east and Europe, where their descendents eventually populated much of the Baltic area and Eastern Europe. Evidence of the reverence with which hemp was viewed by the Scythians appeared in 1993, when Russian archaeologists found the two-thousand-year-old grave of a young Scythian princess in the Siberian Umok plateau. Six horses in full harness were buried with the girl, whose tattooed body was stuffed with fur, moss, and peat. She was dressed in a white silk dress with a crimson wool skirt and white felt stockings. She wore a wooden headdress with a plume of felt. The body was buried in a hollowed larch tree trunk decorated with leather figures of snow leopards and deer and set in a log chamber with a brush, dishes, a mirror, and a small pot containing

■ ■ ■

The Scythians harvested hemp with a curved cutting tool that proved excellent for harvesting other crops as well. The tool is still used in many parts of the world, and it still carries their name—the *scythe*.

■ ■ ■

invaded the Hittite empire about 1000 B.C.E. also wove with true hemp fiber. Excavation of the Phrygian city of Gordion near Ankara, Turkey, unearthed hempen fabrics produced in the late eighth century B.C.E. Cannabis is mentioned in cuneiform tablets dating from 650 B.C.E. (and these are almost certainly copies of much older texts) that were found

cannabis. This discovery is almost identical to the grave of a Scythian chieftain discovered in Siberia in 1929, and perfectly matches descriptions of Scythian burial customs by Herodotus.[13]

Bhang and hashish figure in several tales in the *Book of the Thousand and One Nights,* a collection of Arabic stories compiled between the eleventh and eighteenth centuries. One of the most comical anecdotes is "The Tale of the Hashish Eater," about a beggar who wanders into a bathhouse when no one else is about. He eats some hashish, falls asleep, and dreams that he has a girl in his arms:

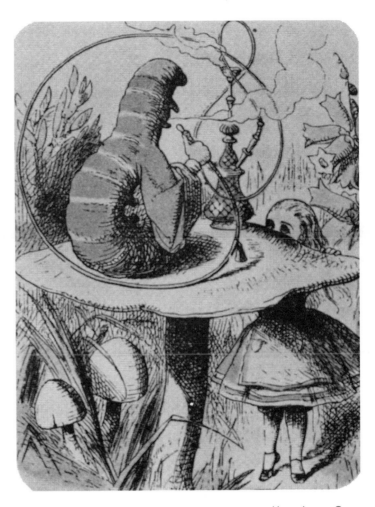

HASHISH APPEARS THROUGHOUT WORLD LITERATURE. HERE, LEWIS CARROLL'S ALICE ENCOUNTERS THE LANGOROUS CATERPILLAR.

> When lo! he heard one saying to him, "Awake, thou ne'er-do-well! The noon-hour is come and thou art still asleep." He opened his eyes and found himself lying on the marge of the cold-water tank, amongst a crowd of people all laughing at him; for his prickle was at point and the napkin had slipped from his middle. So he knew that all this was but a confusion of dreams and an illusion of Hashish and he was vexed and said to him who had aroused him, "Would thou hadst waited till I had put it in!" Then said the folk, "Art thou not ashamed, O Hashish-eater, to be sleeping stark naked with stiff-standing tool?" And they cuffed him till his neck was red. Now he was starving, yet forsooth he had savoured the flavour of pleasure in his dream.[14]

Scheherazade also told "The Tale of the Two Hashish-Eaters," on the 798th night, about a fisherman and a judge who eat hashish

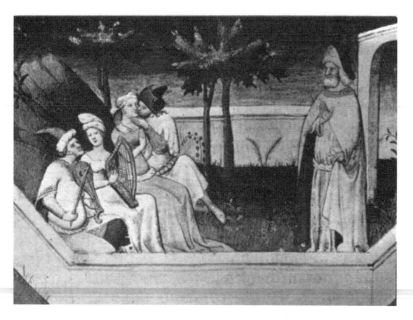

HASAN-IBN-SABAH, LEADER OF THE *HASHASHIN*, WAS RUMORED TO USE HASHISH TO GIVE HIS FOLLOWERS AN EARLY GLIMPSE OF PARADISE.

together and wind up trying to urinate on the sultan and his wazir, who are walking about the city in disguise:

> Next morning, that the jest might be complete, the Sultan called the kadi and his guest before him. . . . Knowing that the Sultan used to walk about the city in disguise, the kadi realised in a flash the identity of his last night's visitors, and fell on his knees, crying: "My lord, my lord, the hashish spake in these indelicacies, not I!" But the fisherman, who by his careful daily taking of the drug was always under its effect, called somewhat sharply: "And what of it? You are in your palace this morning, we were in our palace last night."
>
> "O sweetest noise in all our kingdom," answered the delighted King, "as we are both Sultans of this city, I think you had better henceforth stay with me in my palace. If you can tell stories, I trust that you will at once sweeten our hearing with a chosen one."
>
> "I will do so gladly, as soon as you have pardoned my wazir," replied the fisherman; so the Sultan bade the kadi rise and sent him back forgiven to his duties."[15]

We have hemp to thank for the word *assassin,* a connection that, as we will later see, was used against the plant by etymologically impaired members of Congress in the 1930s. *Assassin* derives from the Arabic *hashashin,* meaning hashish-eater, and owes its origin to a mistake by Marco Polo. While passing through Persia in 1271, Polo heard tales of a cult that lived in a fortress in the mountains and was famed for the murders committed by the fanatical followers of its leader Hasan-ibn-Sabah. The Arabs referred to this cult as *hashashin,* hashish-eaters, but this was a generic derogatory term of the time. Whether the cult actually used hashish is not known. Polo, however, took the name literally and soon after his return to Italy stories of hashish-crazed *assassins* were rampant in Europe.[16]

Africa

By the third millennium B.C.E., the true hemp plant was known in Egypt, where the fibers were used for rope. The ancient Egyptian word for hemp, *smsm t,* occurs in the Pyramid Texts in connection with ropemaking. Pieces of hempen material were found in the tomb of the pharoah Akhenaten (Amenophis IV) at el-Amarna, and pollen on the mummy of Ramses II (circa 1200 B.C.E.) has been identified as cannabis. The Ramses III Papyrus (A. 26) offered an opthalmic prescription containing *smsm t,* and the Ebers Papyrus gave "a remedy to cool the uterus," an enema, and a poultice to an injured toenail, each containing *smsm t.*[17]

Hemp was used in the construction of the pyramids, not only to pull blocks of limestone, but also in the quarries, where the dried fiber was pounded into cracks in the rock, then wetted. As the fiber swelled, the rock broke.

Sir W. Flinders Petrie found a large mat made of palm fiber tied with hemp cordage at el-Amarna, and other digs have unearthed hempen grave clothes of the Badarian, Predynastic, Pan, and Roman periods.

The Punic people who built Carthage in North Africa dominated the Mediterranean Sea from the eleventh to the eighth century B.C.E. and continued as a lesser power until the Romans destroyed them during the three Punic Wars in the third and second centuries B.C.E. A Punic warship found off the coast of Sicily yielded a large quantity of hemp stems; archaeologists speculated that hemp was rationed to the oarsmen, who chewed on it for mild relief from fatigue. Hemp also was used as caulking in ships' hulls, and of course for rope.[18]

Although there is no archaeological evidence that the early Egyptians knew of the psychotropic effects of *smsm t* (hemp), and they did not use hemp fiber to any significant extent, the consumption of cannabis for spiritual reasons or for pleasure eventually became common throughout Africa.

Hashish was known in all the Arab lands, but among one religious sect, the Sufis, it became a part of the religion itself, much as bhang and ganja had among the Hindus. The Sufis—so named because they wore wool *(suf)* for penance—diverged from other Moslems in their belief that

The Hippies of the Arab World

Frustrated by the religious and political climate, a generation breaks away from society. It rejects materialism and desires to live a simple, communal life closer to spiritual truth. The members of this movement dress differently from their peers and embrace cannabis as a catalyst for communion. Because of their differences, and because they do not work, they are reviled by the dominant culture, which views cannabis as the cause of their "downfall."

Sound familiar? The group described above is not the hippies, and the society is not the United States of the late 1960s. Rather, flash back a thousand years to the Sufis, a group Ernest Abel in *Marijuana: The First Twelve Thousand Years* calls "the hippies of the Arab world." According to Abel,

[Sufism] represented a counterculture within the Arab community in the same way that the hippies of the 1960s represented an ideological and behavioral counterculture within American society. Both were peopled by "dropouts" who rejected the dominant economic system in favor of communal living and sharing of material goods. Both had their symbols. For the hippies, it was long hair and beads; for the Sufi, garments made of wool.

Since neither the hippie nor the Sufi had any interest in advancing himself in society or in economic gain, both were looked down upon by the Establishment in their respective eras as being lazy and worthless. In many cases, their behavior was attributed to the effect of drugs. More than intriguing, the dominant drug in both countercultures was made from cannabis. For the hippie, it was marijuana; for the Sufi, hashish. . . . Both marijuana and hashish were accused of sapping the user's energy, thereby robbing him of his willingness to work. This "amotivational syndrome," as it is presently called, was regarded as a threat to the dominant culture since it undermined the work ethic.[20]

What is most striking in Abel's comparison is the fact that, in both cases, cannabis was a central player in an ideological paradigm shift. More than any other psychotropic substance, hemp has been associated with philosophical, sociological, and spiritual realities, rather than simple escapism.

spiritual enlightenment could not be taught or gleaned through rational perception, but only in states of altered consciousness. One method of achieving this entranced state was by the use of hashish. Because of their hashish use, their ascetic ways, and because they came primarily from the lower classes, the Sufis were ostracized by other Arabs. Still, they had strengthened the connection between hashish and Arab spirituality, a connection that remains to this day.[19]

As the hippies of the 1960s were mirrored by the Sufis of the middle ages, so the war on drugs by current world powers has its predecessors in history. Most notorious of these forerunners is Cairo's 125-year crusade to purge itself of hashish. In 1253 the streets of Cairo were filled with Sufis, and consequently filled with hashish. Hemp grew throughout Cafour, a garden in the middle of the city. The authorities decided the situation was out of hand, and every hemp plant in Cafour was destroyed in a huge bonfire that was visible for miles.

As any observer of the modern drug wars could have predicted, this only drove the production of hemp outside the city. Farmers happily supplied Cairo with its hashish until 1324, when once again the government attempted to separate its citizens from their hashish. For thirty days troops were sent into the fields to destroy every hemp plant they could find. But the city soon learned that, while it might be able to control what grew in its gardens, the countryside was too wide and varied and growing hemp was too easy and too lucrative.

In 1378 Cairo took the next step, an ominous one from our perspective: the torture and murder of its citizens. Under orders from Soudan Sheikhoumi, the emir of Joneima, the farmers of *qinnab* were hunted down and executed or imprisoned. The known users were rounded up and had their teeth yanked out with tongs by soldiers before horrified citizens who had assembled nearby. Hashish use continues, of course, to the present day.[21]

Many North African people smoke kif, which they carry in a *mottoni* (pouch) with two or four pockets. Each compartment contains a different grade of kif, which is offered to guests according to the degree of respect or friendship due to them. Kif is smoked in *chquofa*, clay pipes designed for the purpose. An Arabic proverb asserts that "a pipeful of kif before breakfast gives a man the strength of a hundred camels in the courtyard." Another proverb warns, "Kif is like fire—a little warms, a lot burns,"[22] and the *Aqrabadhin of Al-Samarqandi*, an early Arabic medical formulary, recommends hemp seed as a "purging clyster" (enema) to be administered in cases of cold colic.[23]

The earliest archaeological proof of hemp-smoking in Africa outside of Egypt comes from an Ethiopian site near Lake Tana dated to 1320: two ceramic pipe bowls there contained traces of cannabis. The cultivation of hemp (now called *dagga*) spread southward, but the practice of smoking was forgotten along the way and not learned again until the Dutch arrived with their pipes in the seventeenth century. Previously the Hottentots and other tribes had eaten only the leaves, and the pipe was a welcome addition to their cultures; its use spread rapidly and took many forms. Most common were "earth pipes," small holes in the ground that were filled with a mixture of dried *dagga* and smoldering dung. The smokers placed their mouths over the holes and inhaled.[24]

Other tribes developed much more sophisticated techniques. The explorer A. T. Bryant wrote of the Zulus:

> Every Zulu *kraal* had a few hemp-plants growing inside its outer fence for smoking purposes. It was known as *iNtsangu*. . . . Oft of an afternoon one might hear the soft deep boom of the signal-horn

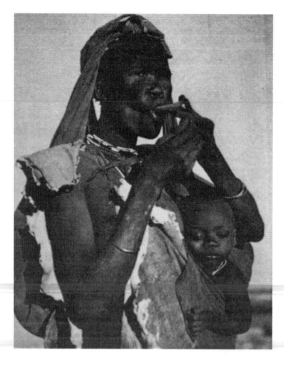

KUNG WOMAN IN SOUTH AFRICA SMOKING *DAGGA*.

of various minor craftsmen—how the maker of smoking-horns (*iGudu*) polished his cow or kudu horn, or carved his hemp-holder (*iMbiza*) out of a nicely carved and polished jade-like soapstone.[25]

Europe

The Scythians carried hemp from Asia through Greece and Russia into Europe, and later Arabs brought hemp from Africa into Spain and other ports of entry on the Mediterranean Sea. Thanks to their love of the nutritious seed, birds also did their unwitting part to spread hemp's global cultivation.

Hesychius reported that Thracian women made sheets of hemp. Moschion (circa 200 B.C.E.) left record of the use of hemp ropes by the tyrant Hiero II, who outfitted the flagship *Syracusia* and others of his fleet with rope made from the superior cannabis cultivated in Rhodanus (the Rhone River Valley). Other Greek city-states obtained much of their hemp from Colchis on the Black Sea. The first-century Greek physician Pedacius Dioscorides described *kannabis emeros* (female) and *agria* (male) in *De Materia Medica* (3:165, 166):

wafting over the veld. This was an invitation by some lonely man to all and sundry to come and keep him company with the hubble-bubble. . . . The hubble-bubble (*iGudu*) was . . . a hollow cow's horn (in the better brands, that of a kudu antelope), finely pared and polished, and used for hemp-smoking. It was fitted with a reed stem (*isiTukulu*), inserted at an acute angle half-way down its side, and carrying on its tip a small bowl (*iMbiza*), the size of an egg. . . . We deem it hardly of sufficient importance to go further into the details of the less significant trades

Kannabis emeros . . . is a plant of much use in this life for ye twistings of very strong ropes, it bears leaves like to the Ash, of a bad scent, long stalks, empty, a round seed, which being eaten of much doth quench geniture, but being juiced when it is green is good for the pains of the ears.

Kannabis agria . . . The root being sodden, and so laid on hath ye force to assuage inflammations and to dissolve Oedemata, and to disperse ye obdurate matter about ye joints. Ye bark also of this, is fitting for ye twining of ropes.[26]

The Roman empire consumed great quantities of hemp fiber, much of which was imported from the Babylonian city of Sura. The cities of Alabanda, Colchis, Cyzicus, Ephesus, and Mylasa also were major centers of hemp industry. Cannabis was not a major crop in early Italy, but the seed was a common food. Carbonized hemp seeds were found in the ruins of Pompeii, buried by the eruption of Mount Vesuvius in the year 79.[27]

Pausanius, in the second century B.C.E., was possibly the first Roman writer to mention hemp; he notes that it was grown in Elide. A surviving fragment of the satirist Lucilius (from about 100 B.C.E.) also mentions the plant. During the reign of Augustus, Lucius Columella gave instructions for the sowing of hemp in *Res Rustica* (II vii.1 and II xii.21). Caius Plinius the Elder (23–79 C.E.) wrote at length about hemp in his *Natural History*. Pliny also reproduced a fragment from the writings of Democritus describing some preparations and effects of cannabis. The Greek physician Galen (about 130–200 C.E.) observed that the Romans ate cannabis pastries at their banquets *cum aliis tragematis*, to promote hilarity.

The Italians called hemp (or *canappa*) *quello delle cento operazioni*, "substance of a hundred operations," because it required so many processes to prepare the fibers for use. The Venetians eventually came to dominate the Italian hemp industry, instituting a craft union and the Tana, a state-operated spinning factory with demanding production standards. The Venetian senate declared that "the security of our galleys and ships and similarly of our sailors and capital" rests on "the manufacture of cordage in our home of the Tana." Statutes required that all Venetian ships be rigged only with the best quality of hemp rope. From its advantageous location, the superior Venetian fleet controlled Mediterranean shipping until the city was conquered by Napoléon in 1797.[28]

• • •

Classical Cannabis

Numerous ancient Greek and Roman writers make literary reference to hemp. A sampling of the formidable list includes Leo Africanus, who writes in *The History and Description of Africa* about the Lhasis potation in Tunisia; Alus Gellus, writing in *Noctes Atticae*; Caius Plinius the Elder in *Natural History*; Galen in *De Facultatibus Alimentorum*; Cato in *De Re Rustica*; Gaius Catullus in *Codex Veronensis*; Herodotus in *The Histories*; Lucius Columella in *Res Rustica*; Pedacius Dioscorides in *De Materia Medica*; and Plutarch in *Of the Names of Mountains and Rivers*. Theophrastus wrote of the *dendromalache*, "the herb tree." Among the other classical writers who took notice of hemp are Aetius, Democritus, Cinegius, Hesychius, Lucilius, Moschion, Pausanius, Strabo, and Titus Livius.

■ ■ ■

The Romans helped spread hemp through Europe, although the plant was well known there already. A sixth-century B.C.E. tomb at Wilmersdorf (Brandenburg) offered up an urn containing sand and an assortment of plant fragments, including hemp seeds and pericarps, when it was excavated by German archaeologist Herman Busse in 1896.[29] The Vikings relied on hemp as rope, sailcloth, caulking, and fishline and nets for their daring voyages; thus, they may have introduced cannabis to the east coast of North America. Hemp seed was found in the remains of Viking ships that must have been built about 850. Equally ancient retting pits have been discovered in Denmark. In 1753 the Swedish botanist Carl von Linne, or Linnaeus (1707–1778), classified hemp as *Cannabis sativa* in his *Species Plantarum* and described the resin as a narcotic. Linnaeus cultivated cannabis on his windowsill in order to closely study its sexuality.

Farther to the south, the path of hemp had traveled with the West Germanic people known as Franks, who entered the Roman provinces in 253 C.E. and eventually occupied most of Gaul. When the crypt of the Frankish Queen Arnemunde (who died in 570) was unearthed, she was found surrounded by spectacular treasure and wearing a silk dress and gold jewelry. The body was draped in hemp cloth, showing that the humble plant was held in high esteem.

Hemp figured in the fire festivals of several European countries. In the French Ardennes it was believed vital that the women be intoxicated on the night of the first Sunday in Lent if the hemp were to grow tall that season. In medieval Swabia, in southwest Germany, the nubile men and women leaped hand-in-hand over a bonfire crying "Grow, that the hanf may be three ells high!" It was thought that those who made the jump would not suffer from backache when they reaped the crop, and the parents of those young people who jumped highest would enjoy the most abundant harvest. If a farmer failed to add anything to the bonfire, his crops in general were cursed and his hemp in particular was doomed to failure.[30]

French farmers, too, were wont to dance during the Lenten carnival so their *chanvre* would grow tall. In the Vosges Mountain region, people danced on the roofs of their houses on Twelfth Day, the Epiphany, for the same purpose. When sowing hemp seed, farmers would pull up their pants as far as possible in the belief that the plants would grow precisely to the height of their britches. Other men jumped as high as they could in the field, believing that this activity made the hemp grow taller. In the Bean Festival of Lorraine farmers made predictions about the hemp crop by comparing heights of the king and queen. If the king was taller than the queen, then the male hemp would grow higher than the female, and vice versa.[31]

The brilliant French priest, scholar, lawyer, and physician Francois Rabelais (1483–1553) devotes three chapters of his great satire, *Gargantua and Pantagruel*, to a botanical description of "Pantagruelion" (his coinage for hemp). He gives a panegyric account of its many virtues; from its daily uses to the way it enabled ships to have "leaped over the Atlantic Ocean, swept past both tropics, vaulted down under the torrid zone, and measured the whole zodiac, frisking along under the equinoxes, with both the poles dancing on their horizon."

> Just as [the drink] Plantagruel has been the ideal and symbol of all joyous perfection . . . in Pantagruelion, too, I see such enormous potential, such energy, so many perfections, so many admirable accomplishments, that [without] its powers . . . our kitchens would

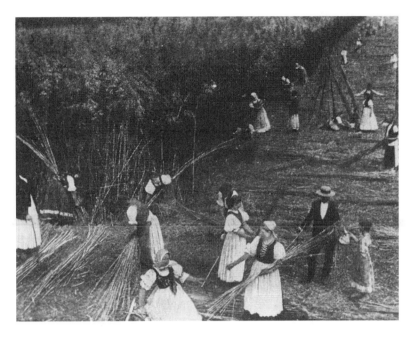

TURN-OF-THE-CENTURY HEMP HARVEST.

> be unspeakable, our tables disgusting, even if they were covered with all sorts of exquisite delicacies—and our beds would offer no delight. . . . Without Pantagruelion, millers could not carry wheat to their mills, or bring back flour. Without Pantagruelion, how would lawyers ever manage to bring their briefs to court? How, without it, would you ever carry plaster into workshops? Or draw water from wells? Without Pantagruelion, . . . the noble art of printing would surely perish. What would we use to make window coverings? How would we ring our church bells? The priests of Isis are adorned with Pantagruelion, as are

the statue-bearing priests around the world, and all human beings when they first come into this world. All the wool-bearing trees of India, the cotton vines of Tylos, in the Persian Sea, like the cotton plants of Arabia, and the cotton vines of Malta do not adorn as many people as this one herb. It covers armies against rain and cold, . . . It shapes and makes possible boots, and half-boots, and sea boots, spats, and laced boots, and shoes, and dancing shoes, slippers, and hob boots. Pantagruelion strings bows, pulls crossbows tight, and makes slings. And just as if it were a sacred herb, like verbena, worshipped by the souls of the dead, corpses are never buried without it. . . . By the use of this herb, which captures and holds the waves of the air, great ships are sent hither and thither . . . nations which nature seemed to keep hidden away, obscure, impenetrable, unknown, have now come to us, and we to them— something even the birds could not do, no matter how light their feathers or what powers of flight they are given.[32]

Although Rabelais claimed the glories of hemp for France, the Moors had founded Europe's first paper factory in 1150, utilizing hemp cultivated around the city of Xativa (as in sativa) in Alicante province, Spain. Additional Moorish hemp-milling operations were established in Toledo and Valencia. The other countries of Europe soon followed suit, producing hempen rag paper in the same manner as had the Chinese a millenium earlier. Printers began publishing the Bible on hemp paper as soon as Gutenburg invented movable type in the fifthteenth century.[33]

When Napoléon Bonaparte invaded Egypt in 1798, thousands of his soldiers, faced with the unavailablity of alcohol in the Moslem world, immediately took to the use of hashish. Previously, hashish had been just an exotic foreign word known to well-read Europeans. Suddenly it became a real experience that threatened military discipline. In October 1800 Napoléon proclaimed, "It is forbidden in all of Egypt to use certain Moslem beverages made with hashish or likewise to inhale the smoke from seeds of hashish."[34]

Unfortunately for Napoléon, the French expedition was accompanied by 175 scholars, a group never known for their discipline. They enjoyed hashish so much as to send a quantity of it to France for their colleagues to study, and a scientific report on solvent extracts of hashish appeared in

1803. When the eminent Silvestre de Sacy addressed the Institute of France on the subject in 1809, he announced that the word "assassin" was derived from hashish. On such authority, belief in the use of hashish by a secret order of Moslem terrorists called Assassins was certified and once again became well established in the popular literature of the period.

Humble hemp was instrumental in the downfall of Napoléon. In 1812 Bonaparte invaded Russia with the ill-considered intent of devastating her hemp crops to inflict punishment on Czar Alexander I, and to ruin England's navy, which without hemp would have no sails or rope. The Czar had violated the 1807 Treaty of Tilset by continuing to sell hemp to England through American traders (many of whom were strongly "impressed" by the Royal Navy to serve as a "flag of convenience" for British interests). The Russian winter utterly decimated Napoléon's mighty army, but hemp has continued to flourish on the steppes.[36]

Pieces of hemp rope found in the well of a Roman fort—on the Antonine wall at Bar Hill in Dunbartonshire—indicate that the Romans introduced cannabis to the British Isles at least by 180 C.E. The plant was not cultivated and retted in Britain until about 400, however, when hemp and flax were first grown at Old Buckenham Mere.[37]

The Saxons who occupied Britain about 600 C.E. also cultivated hemp and incorporated it into their medical literature. *The Commonplace Book* (LXIII C., folio 147a) gives a "Rite for Salve, Partly Irish" that contains hemp, placed high on the list of fifty-nine ingredients in a sustained alliteration of plant names that is unique in Anglo-Saxon literature:

> *As a holy salve:*
> *"Shall [serve] betonys and bennet,*
> *and hindheal and hemp, raspberry*
> *   and ironhard*
> *sage and savine, bishopwort and*
> *   rosemary . . .", etc.*[38]

Although the sixteenth-century demonologist Jean Wier warned that hemp caused one to lose one's speech, to laugh without control, and to have magnificent visions, and in the seventeenth century demonologist Giovanni De Ninault named hemp flowers and the oil of hemp seed as principal ingredients of Satanic unguents, peasants continued to believe in the magical power of hemp, and practiced their traditions as ever. On Saint John's Eve, farmers would pick flowers from

---

■■■

If hemp was already a familiar fiber crop in Europe, why were its psychoactive properties unknown? According to the nineteenth-century scholar Baron Ernst von Bibra:

> The Indian hemp plant . . . has very different chemical properties than the European plant. It contains substances that do not mature in our colder climate, or develop only in small amounts. In short, it is a situation similar to that of the poppy plant, which yields only small amounts of opium here in Europe, or of the rose, from which hardly a drop of rose oil can be extracted, whereas large quantities are extracted from it in the Orient.[35]

Later studies have shown that the psychoactive resin produced by hemp protects its upper flowers and leaves from moisture loss in hot or desert climates.

■■■

some of their hemp plants and feed them to their livestock to protect the animals from evil and sickness. Hemp was a common and popular folk remedy, used to treat toothaches, to facilitate childbirth, to reduce convulsions, fevers, inflammations, and swollen joints, and to cure rheumatism and jaundice. Cannabis was found worthy of honorable mention as a healing plant in several medieval herbals, including those by William Turner, Mattioli, and Dioscobas Taberaemontanus.[39]

The Conquest of the Seas

By the fifteenth century the struggle for power in Western Europe had become a struggle to dominate the seas. Spain, Holland, and England were envious of the riches from the Orient reaching Venice via the silk road, but realized that their location excluded them from the land trade routes. The only way to get a piece of the action was to bypass these routes entirely by establishing a sea trade that led right to their door. This meant they needed hemp, and lots of it—only the long, strong fibers of hemp could produce canvas sails and thick rope tough enough to weather the punishing

journey to the Orient. Without hemp, Europe's ships would be stuck hugging its gentle coasts.

The Dutch took an early lead in hemp production because of superior technology and equipment. In Holland, windmills (themselves powered by hemp sails) provided power to crush the stalks of *hennep*, an enormous saving of manual labor that enabled the Dutch to produce vast quantities of *canefas* ("canvas," from the Latin *cannabis*) and rope that aided their ascendance as a powerful seafaring nation. The Dutch used advanced techniques of bleaching hemp and linen; in 1756 they introduced dilute sulphuric acid to the six month process for retting, washing, heating, and watering, and cut the time required in half.[40] Still, Holland faced the same problem as their western rivals: they could not grow nearly enough hemp to meet their needs. The Dutch traded with the Scandinavian and Baltic countries, and especially with Russia and Italy, for their provisions of the strategic material.

Because of their island location, the British were in an even more compromising position than Holland or Spain, since they depended on hemp to maintain their naval power as well as their mercantile interests. As early as

1533, King Henry VIII required all farmers to cultivate one quarter acre of hemp or flax for every sixty acres of land under tillage. Queen Elizabeth repeated the edict in 1563, but farmers were so reluctant to grow the crop that the order was repealed in 1593. With arable soil at a premium, British farmers were not enthusiastic about growing hemp; it did not pay well (even with the incentive of bounties granted by the Crown) and farmers did not know much about the plant's requirements and subtleties.[41] The conservative farmers could not be confident of success with the crop, and most could not afford to experiment. They did not appreciate the labor involved in retting hemp, nor the foul smell, described starkly in a 1580 volume titled *Five Hundred Points of Good Husbandrie*:

> Now pluck up they hempe, and go
>   beat out the seed,
> and afterward water it as ye see
>   need.
> But not in the river where cattle
>   should drink,
> for poisoning them and the people
>   with stinke.[42]

In *How to Use All Land Profitably* (1607), J. Norton opines on behalf of this misunderstood crop, ad-

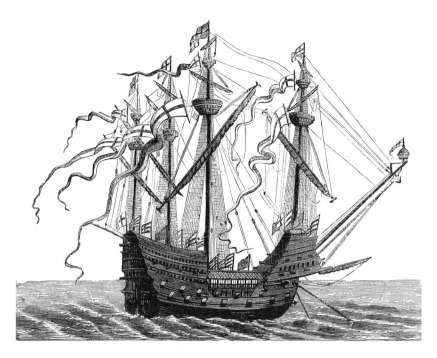

THE *GREAT HARRY,* PART OF THE HEMPEN FLEET OF HENRY VIII. ILLUSTRATION COURTESY OF JIM HARTER.

monishing that "many crofts, tofts, pightles, pingles, and other small quillets of land, about farm houses and tenements, are suffered to lie together idle, some overgrown with . . . unprofitable weeds, which are fat and fertile, where, if the farmer would use the means, would grow sundry commodities, as hemp. . . . The hemp is of great use in a farmer's house, . . . not only for cordage for shipping, but also for linen, and other necessaries about a house."[43]

Despite its utility, hemp seemed always to be falling short of its economic potential. When the Eastland merchant venture floundered early in the seventeenth century, King James I asked the Commission on Trade why the dressing of hemp was no longer handled by English laborers who needed the work, and he was told:

> Our Eastland Merchants in former tymes did lade their Shipps with Hempe and Flax rough dressed in great Quantities, which did not onlie helpe them much in their Retornes, but did also set great Numbers of our People on work with dressing the same, and converting the same into Lynnen Cloth, which kind of Trade we understand is of late almost given over, by bringing in of Hemp and Flax ready dressed, and that for the most part by Strangers.[44]

In 1651 the London hemp dressers petitioned Charles I, demanding that the importation of already-dressed hemp from the Netherlands be "prohibited, restrained, and forbidden." The industry knew it was facing the same fate that had come to dressers of flax: competition from the Dutch was to leave them "utterly decayed and brought to beggary."[45]

Only a decade later, in fact, there were not enough hemp dressers available; so in 1663 the Crown passed the Act for Encour-

aging the Manufactures of Making Linen Cloth and Tapestry, in which the British invited alien workers "to set up and exercise the trade, occupation or mystery of breaking, hickling, or dressing of hemp or flax," enticing them with an offer of full citizenship within three years of establishing themselves in England. Local manufacture could not keep pace with the British demand for hemp, and in 1696 Ireland was permitted to export yarn and cloth made from hemp and flax duty-free to England.[46]

Despite all her efforts, England remained dependent on Russia for as much as 97 percent of her hemp. Not only was this economically crippling, it also placed England in constant jeopardy; all an unfriendly power had to do was cut off her hemp supply, and England would be at their mercy. (Napoléon would later attempt to do just this.) Desperate to safeguard her independence, and having had no luck doing so at home or elsewhere in Europe, England shifted her gaze westward.

For indeed the Atlantic was no longer the beast it had always seemed. Hemp and some intrepid navigators had seen to that. Christopher Columbus had ridden eighty tons of hemp rigging and vast stretches of hemp canvas across the Atlantic in 1492. The

Spanish had found poorly defended kingdoms of vast wealth in the new world, and the thought of pillaging a few northern kingdoms appealed to England as well. The Mayflower, also powered by hemp, had made the crossing, and reports were that hemp grew beautifully in the new world, better than it ever had in Europe.[47]

And so they came. Hemp's story and mankind's story had twisted together for millenia, but never before had their expansion been so interdependent, and never would anything in their mutual past be as bizarre as the twists and turns that lay ahead. For by beckoning their ships to go farther and faster, and with its natural affinity for the soils and climates of the new world, hemp seemed to almost usher civilization into the next great development on the world stage—that noble, tragic, contradictory experiment called America.

5

THE
PATRIOTIC
CROP

Natives, Explorers,
and Colonists

The Vikings depended on hemp for their sails and rope, and they
probably carried hemp seed with them and planted it when they
visited North America about a thousand years ago. Sailors usually carried
supplies of seeds with them to provide the necessities of life in case of
shipwreck. *Cannabis* was already in North America in prehistoric times,
possibly brought from China by explorers, drifting shipwrecks, and birds
migrating across the Bering Strait to the west coast of the continent.[1]

Some of the earliest evidence of hemp in North America is associated
with the ancient Mound Builders of the Great Lakes and Mississippi Valley. Hundreds of clay pipes, some containing cannabis residue and
wrapped in hemp cloth, were found in the so-called Death Mask Mound
of the Hopewell Mound Builders, who lived about 400 B.C.E. in modern
Ohio. In his 1891 study, *Prehistoric Textile Art of Eastern United States,*
Smithsonian Institute ethnologist W. H. Holmes describes the recovery of
large pieces of hemp fabric at one site in Morgan County, Tennessee: the
"friends of the dead deposited with the body not only the fabrics worn
during life but a number of skeins of the fiber from which the fabrics
were probably made. This fiber has been identified as that of the *Cannabis sativa,* or wild hemp."[2]

Nearly two millennia after the age of the Mound Builders, European explorers seemed reassured by meeting up with a familiar plant upon their arrival in an alien "new world." The Florentine Giovanni da Verrazano wrote thoughtfully of the natives encountered during a French expedition to Virginia in 1524: "We found those folkes to be more white than those that we found before, being clad with certain leaves that hang on boughs of trees, which they sewe together with threds of wilde hemp."[3] The French explorer Jacques Cartier also reported seeing wild hemp during each of his three journeys to Canada between 1535 and 1541. His last report enthused that "the land groweth full of Hempe which groweth of it selfe, which is as good as possibly may be seene, and as strong." Later, Samuel de Champlain mentioned in 1605 that the natives used "wild hemp" to tie their bone fishhooks.

The first European colonists used wild hemp when they arrived in America. There was not enough of it, however, and labor was in short supply too. Food crops, especially corn, were the first priority, and the colonists were not eager to grow hemp, although the seed is excellent food.

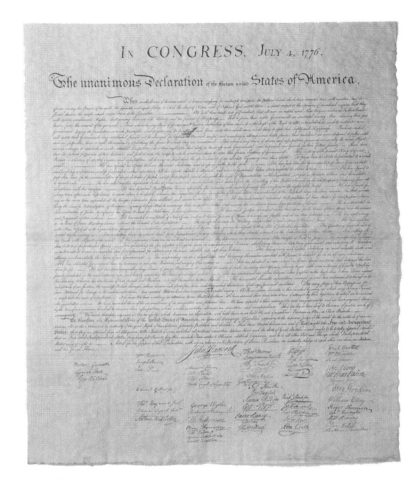

THE DECLARATION OF INDEPENDENCE. IT WAS THE SUMMER OF 1776 AND HEMP MADE HISTORY.

But the European motherland wanted hemp, and in service to France Quebec colony minister Jean Talon simply confiscated all the thread the colonists possessed and forced them to buy it back from him with hemp. He loaned the necessary seed to the farmers, who were required to reimburse Talon with fresh hemp seed from their harvest.[4]

The first American ropewalk for manufacturing hemp rope was built in Salem in 1635. Boston merchants organized to persuade ropemaker John Harrison to migrate from England in 1642, and gave him a lifelong monopoly. By 1770 there were fourteen ropewalks in Boston, and at least one in almost every coastal town. Benedict Arnold destroyed the strategic Public Rope Walk in Warwick, Virginia, when he led British forces up the Jones River in April 1781. The spectacle of a large rope factory inspired the poet Henry Wadsworth Longfellow to write "The Ropewalk" in 1854:

In that building, long and
*   low,*
With its windows all a-row,
Like the port-holes of a hulk,
Human spiders spin and
*   spin,*
Backwards down their
*   thread so thin,*
Dropping, each a hempen
*   thread . . ."*

■ ■ ■

Hemp cultivation was deemed mandatory for English colonists as well. The Puritans grew hemp at Jamestown in keeping with their 1607 contract with the Virginia Company. Virginia governor Sir Thomas Dale brought with him instructions to plant a communal garden in which to experiment with hemp and flax. By 1616, the Puritans were able to claim of their flax and hemp that there was "none better in England or Holland."[5] But however vital hemp and flax were to the economy, colonists preferred to grow tobacco. Tobacco prices were almost always higher, supported by Europeans already hooked on nicotine, and tobacco was less labor-intensive. Despite the overwhelming demand for hemp, only when the tobacco market went through periodic crashes would tobacco farmers "rediscover" hemp, and they always went back to tobacco after the market recovered. In response the Virginia Company issued a directive in 1619 that every Jamestown colonist was to "set 100 plants and the governor to set 5000" hemp plants. In the same year, the Virginia General Assembly also required the colonists to grow "both English and Indian hemp." Gabriel Wisher was assigned a budget of 100 pounds with which to hire several skilled Swedish and Polish hemp dressers and entice them (with ten pounds each) to emigrate to America.[11-13]

Some Massachusetts colonists led by Thomas Morton founded the Merrymount trading settlement, where they began to view the world in a new way, inspired by smoking hemp in the peace pipe with natives. Their bonfire and Maypole parties eventually evoked the rage of the Puritans, who burned down the outpost and sent Morton to an English prison.

Mandatory hemp cultivation continued in later years and in other areas of the New World. In 1637 the General Court at Hartford, Connecticut, ordered all families to plant one teaspoonful of hemp seed. Massachusetts did likewise in 1639. The General Assembly of Connecticut repeated its order in 1640, insisting that the colonists sow hemp "that we might in time have supply of linen cloth among ourselves."

Several colonies passed legal-tender laws by which certain manufactures, particularly hemp, flax, and tar, could be used to pay debts and taxes. Hemp was so valuable and necessary to the British economy that in 1662 Parliament authorized Virginia governor William Berkeley to offer a bounty of two pounds of tobacco per pound of finished hemp, and other colonies offered similar enticements. By 1690 there was enough hemp, flax, and cotton available in North America to supply a paper industry. The first paper mill in America was established in Pennsylvania by the firm of Rittenhouse, and others followed suit.

The success of hemp cultivation impressed those who witnessed crops at their peak. The Dutch farmer Antoine Le Page du Pratz, who came to America to act as overseer of French plantations near the present site of New Orleans and who was familiar with true hemp, wrote in his journal in 1719: "I ought not to omit to take notice, that hemp grows naturally on the lands adjoining to the lakes on the west of the Mississippi. The stalks are as thick as one's finger, and about six feet long. They are quite like ours in the wood, the leaf and the rind."[6]

Colonial governments encouraged hemp production with varying degrees of severity and success. The 1720–1722 sessions of the Connecticut General Assembly approved a bounty of four shillings per "gross hundred" of partially processed hemp to encourage its continued cultivation, while Virginia continued to pass laws designed to compel land-

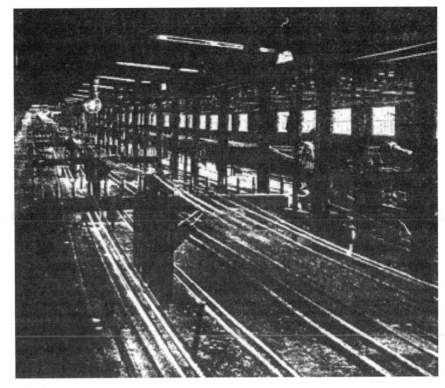

EARLY TWENTIETH-CENTURY ROPEWALK.

owners to produce the crop, fining farmers who did not comply. Others states were more diplomatic: South Carolina's legislature voted in 1733 to pay a salary to Richard Hall to educate the public about the benefits of hemp and the need for hemp and its cultivation. He was hired to write a book on the subject, promote the hemp industry for three years, and travel to Holland to procure good hemp seed. Local governments may well have been hoping that this crop would provide economic stability for the new colonies. Jared Eliot stressed the potential of hemp as America's trademark product in his *Essays Upon Field Husbandry in New England* which appeared in 1739: "England is possessed of the Woolen Trade, and Ireland of the Linnen Trade; so that this Hemp Trade lies open to us, which may in time become our Staple for Returns Home; and so bring the Balance of Trade to be in our Favour, which has always as yet been against us." Unfortunately for the colonies, the crown was not interested in having them develop a "trademark product."

A ban on spinning and weaving was a cornerstone of seventeenth-century colonial policy designed to foster dependence on England. The motherland demanded raw goods to nourish her own economies and labor forces, and colonists were expected to export fiber and then buy back finished products at value-added prices. By the eighteenth century, however, English merchants were so overstocked with dry goods that they were dumping linens on the American market at fire-sale prices. This might have simply cemented colonial dependency on fabrics from the home state, but what happened instead is that professional spinners and weavers from Ireland began arriving in Massachusetts in 1718 in waves that peaked in 1745. The immigrants introduced improved modes of "spinningwork" that produced more cloth from flax and hemp. New England women began to hold spinning bees, and by the time of the War for Independence from the British Crown they were self-sufficient enough to boycott English fabric products. The early American paper industry relied mainly on hemp, linen, and cotton rags for raw material, and benefited greatly from this increased domestic production.

Throughout the revolutionary era, helpful manuals to aid the would-be hemp farmer continued to appear, often at the behest of colonial governments eager to erect stable, self-sufficient economies with this versatile crop as their foundation. The Massachusetts House of Representatives in 1765 commissioned *A Treatise of Hemp-Husbandry* from Edmund Quincy, who summarized:

> It is presumed none will be at a loss to determine, that the two most important materials which the Inhabitants of these Colonies should be principally encouraged in the growth of, are Flax and Hemp, being the most extensively useful of any which can be so easily and generally produced in North America.

In the introduction to his *Observations on the Raising and Dressing of Hemp,* written in 1777, Edward Antil declared, "Hemp is one of the most profitable productions the earth furnishes in northern climates; as it employs a great number of poor people in a very advantageous manner, if its manufacture is carried on properly: It . . . becomes worthy of the serious attention . . . of every trading man, who truly loves his country."[7]

With the Revolution at hand, the prominent Virginia landowner and politician Robert "King" Carter anticipated in 1774 that his tobacco "next summer will be in little demand," and he instructed his foreman, "in place of tobacco—hemp and flax will be grown." Mandatory cultivation laws were passed "as a preparation for war. . . . Each tithable . . . is bound to deliver every year one pound each of dressed hemp and flax or two pounds of either . . . under oath that it was of his own growth."[8] A revolution is fought on more fronts than just the battlefield, and hemp, as the major source of paper in the colonies, was essential for communication. In addition to clothing the revolutionary soldiers and equipping the navy, hemp-paper pamphlets and documents spread the revolution of ideas through the colonies and helped establish the desire for independence in colonists' minds. By the time Thomas Paine exhorted his fellows to fight for freedom with *Common Sense* in January 1776, he could point out that "in almost every article of defence we abound. Hemp flourishes even to rankness, so that we need not want cordage."[9]

The Founding Fathers

Despite Thomas Paine's confidence, the colonies and the new United States never produced enough hemp to meet their needs. The Founding Fathers nonetheless held out hope for the potential role of hemp in the economy of the new nation. The papers of Alexander Hamilton contain numerous mentions of hemp, and his famous "report on manufactures" of 1791 (written during his term as the first secretary of the U.S. Treasury) contends that hemp is "an article of importance enough to warrant the employment of extraordinary means in its favor."

George Washington and Thomas Jefferson both had firsthand experience with hemp husbandry: as farmer-politicians, they each worked avidly to promote the

> ■ ■ ■
>
> The first and second drafts of the Declaration of Independence were written on Dutch hemp paper in the summer of 1776. The second draft was submitted, agreed upon, then copied onto animal parchment and signed on 2 August 1776.
>
> ■ ■ ■

George Washington

•••

George Washington, a hemp farmer, made these entries in his farm diary in 1765:

May 12/13: Sowed Hemp at Muddy hole by Swamp. Sowed Ditto above the Meadow at Doeg Run.

May 15: Sowed Do. at head of the Muddy H.

May 16: Sowed Hemp at head of the Meadow at Doeg Run & Southwards Houses with the Barel.

May 18: Began to Sow the old Dg. next the Orchard at Muddy hole with the Drill & finished 25 Rows then stopd sowing two fast.

May 20: Sowed 14 Rows more—the drill beg. altered with 1 bushel of seed.

Aug. 7: Began to separate the Male from the Female hemp at Muddy hole—rather too late.

Aug. 9: Abt 6 Oclock put some Hemp in the Rvr. to Rot.

Aug. 15: The English Hemp i.e. the Hemp from the English seed was picked at Muddy hole this day & was ripe. Began to separate Hemp in the Neck.

Aug. 22: Put some Hemp into the Water about 6 Oclock in the afternoon—note this Hemp had been pulled the 8th Instt. & was well dryed, & took it out again the 26th.

Aug. 29: Pulling up the [male] hemp. Was too late for the blossom hemp by three weeks or a month.

Washington wrote to Robert Cary & Co. in London on 20 September 1765 and requested a quotation for what American hemp might bring: "In order thereto you would do me a singular favour in advising of the general price one might expect for good Hemp in your Port watered and prepared according to Act of Parliament, with an estimate of the freight, and all other Incident charges pr. Tonn that I may form some Idea of the profits resulting from the growth." In a letter to Capel and Osgood Hanbury written the same day, he repeated the request. The diary continues:

Sept. 25: Hemp seed seems to be in good order for getting—that is of a proper ripeness—but oblige to desist to pull my fodder.

Oct. 10: Finished pulling Seed Hemp at River Plantation.

Oct. 12: Finished pulling Do. Do. at Doeg Run. Not much, if any, too late for the seed.

Oct. 31: Finished sowing Wheat in Hemp Ground at River Plantation & plowed in a good deal of Shattered Hemp seed—27 bushels in all.[10]

•••

reputation of the crop and to improve its culture. Their interest may not have been entirely commercial: George Washington may well have cultivated some virgin female hemp for medicinal purposes and for occasional recreational smoking. He and Thomas Jefferson, who disliked tobacco, are known to have exchanged gifts of smoking mixtures. Washington reportedly preferred to smoke hemp flowers, although no hard evidence is documented.

In addition to various commercial, medicinal, and recreational uses of hemp, Washington was introduced to the nutritional potential of the herb. In a letter to Dr. James Anderson, dated 26 May 1794, Washington gratefully acknowledges receipt of a sample (presumably dry) of a traditional northern European soup made with hemp seed and millet:

I thank you as well for the Seeds as for the Pamphlets which you had the goodness to send me. The artificial preparation of Hemp, from Silesia [an area between Germany and Poland], is really a curiosity; and I shall think myself much favored in the continuance of your corrispondence. . . .

In the 1790s Washington began to cultivate "Indian hemp,"

the resinous hemp developed in India. (Today the term "Indian hemp" refers to jute, which is not related to *Cannabis sativa,* true hemp. Jute was not introduced to North America until much later.) As a farmer, Washington was well aware of the difference between "common hemp" (*C. sativa*), cultivated for fiber and seeds, and "Indian hemp" (*C. indica*), grown for fiber and resin. On 29 May 1796 he wrote in a letter to William Pearce:

> What was done with the Seed saved from the India Hemp last summer? It ought, all of it, to have been sown again; that not only a stock of seed sufficient for my own purposes might have been raised, but to have disseminated the seed to others; as it is more valuable than the common Hemp.

Throughout the 1790s, Washington's letters to Pearce, his overseer, are preoccupied with the planting, sowing, and especially the saving of seed from this important new stock. "Make the most of it," he urges anxiously, again and again, and suggests sowing on ground where the plants will be most secure from the incursions of rabbits and birds. The instructions in a letter of 5 November 1796 capture his typi-

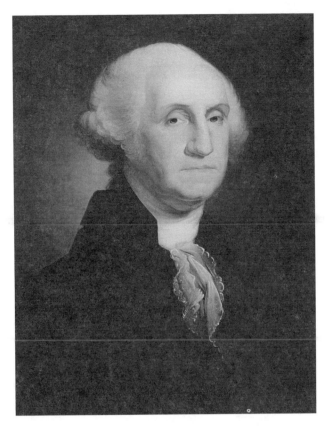

GEORGE WASHINGTON, HEMP FARMER.

cal eagerness about the crop's success: "Let particular care be taken of the India Hemp seed, and as much good grd. allotted for its reception next year as is competent to Sow."

In 1781 the new governor of Virginia, Thomas Jefferson, had reserves of "hemp in the back country" for use as payment for Virginia's military supplies. Virginia's purchasing agent, David Ross, notified Jefferson on 16 May 1781 that the state's delegates

Thomas Jefferson

Thomas Jefferson grew hemp, and he kept a record of his enterprises and thoughts on the matter in his account books, in *Notes on Tobacco*, and other writings.

Hemp. Plough the ground for it early in the fall & very deep, if possible plough it again in Feb. before you sow it, which should be in March. A hand can tend 3 acres of hemp a year. Tolerable ground yields 500 lb. to the acre. You may generally count on 100 lb. for every foot the hemp is over 4 f. high. A hand will break 60 or 70 lb. a day, and even to 150 lb. if it is divided with an overseer, divide it as prepared.

Seed. To make hemp seed, make hills of the form & size of cucumber hills, from 4. to 6. f. apart, in proportion to the strength of the ground. Prick about a dozen seeds into each hill, in different parts of it. When they come up thin them to two. As soon as the male plants have shed their farina, cut them up that the whole nourishment may go to the female plants. Every plant thus ended will yield a quart of seed. A bushel of good brown seed is enough for an acre.[11]

had "no encouragement from Congress . . . in money matters. Tobacco will not do there [in Philadelphia] and we have nothing to depend upon but our hemp." The next month, on 21 June, the Virginia General Assembly put forth a plan to help its impoverished delegates raise money by sending them hemp or tobacco to sell.[12] As was the case for Washington, it was not simply its usefulness as currency that sustained Jefferson's interest in hemp. Jefferson found hemp as an agricultural crop to be superior to tobacco, as

he explained in his farm journal of 16 March 1791, because

The culture [of tobacco] is pernicious. This plant greatly exhausts the soil. Of course, it requires much manure, therefore other productions are deprived of manure, yielding no nourishment for cattle, there is no return for the manure expended. . . . The fact well established in the system of agriculture is that the best hemp and the best tobacco grow on the same kind of soil. The former article is of the first necessity to the commerce and marine, in other words to the wealth and protection of the country. The latter, never useful and sometimes pernicious, derives its estimation from caprice, and its best value from the taxes to which it was formerly exposed. The preference to be given will result from a comparison of them: Hemp employs in its rudest form more labor than tobacco, but being a material for manufactures of various sorts, becomes afterwards the means of support to numbers of people, hence it is to be preferred in a populous country.[13]

Remarkably little has changed since Jefferson's day. Tobacco, as pernicious as ever, continues to cause society unimaginable damage in the forms of death and disease. Its only advantage from a farmer's point of view is the steady demand for it from addicted consumers. And the high tax revenue it generates—a 200-year-old excuse—we now know doesn't begin to pay the health-care costs for which it is clearly responsible.

Jefferson was not fond of flax either. In a letter of December 1815 he argues that "flax is so injurious to our lands and of so scanty produce that I have never attempted it. Hemp, on the other hand, is abundantly productive and will grow forever on the same spot." The breaking and beating of hemp in fiber production was so slow and laborious, however, that Jefferson had given up growing it. "But recently, he continued in the same letter, "a method of removing the difficulty of preparing hemp occurred to me, so simple and so cheap. I modified a threshing machine to turn a very strong hemp-break, much stronger and heavier than those for the hand. By this . . . it is more perfectly beaten than I have ever seen done by hand. . . . I expect that a single horse will do the breaking and beating of ten men." The hemp-break invented by Jefferson received the first U.S. patent, and he estimated that it

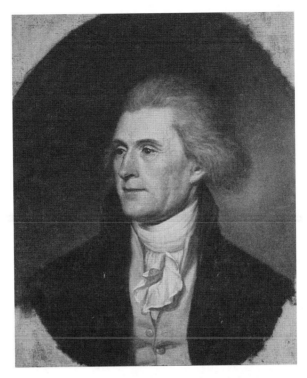

THOMAS JEFFERSON, A MAJOR HEMP PROMOTER, SMUGGLED RARE HEMP SEEDS FROM EUROPE FOR AMERICAN FARMERS.

would cost a person with a threshing machine not more than twelve or fifteen dollars to add the hemp-working device.[14]

Hemp in Nineteenth-Century America

By 1810 Russia had become one of the most important markets for American products. The United States sent 10 percent of its exports, most importantly tobacco,

∎∎∎

The USS *Constitution* carried hemp sails and more than sixty tons of hemp rigging, including an anchor cable nearly two feet in circumference and 720 feet long. The total length of running rigging was more than four miles of soft- and hard-laid hemp.

∎∎∎

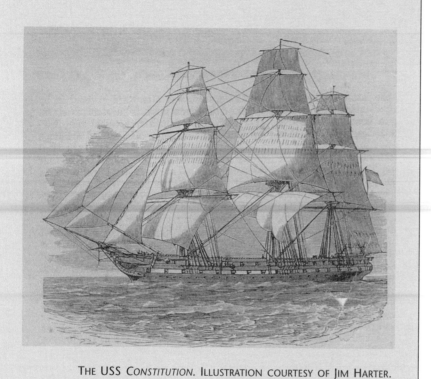

THE USS *CONSTITUTION*. ILLUSTRATION COURTESY OF JIM HARTER.

Quincy Adams, the sixth president of the United States (who had lived in Russia as a young man) wrote a report in 1810 *On the Culture and Preparing of Hemp in Russia*. The entire process of growing, water-retting, breaking, and hackling hemp to prepare the fiber for cloth production required up to two years to complete and deliver to port. This arduous method was only possible because muzhik, or serf labor, was so cheap in Russia. The stalks were hung on racks for two days immediately after harvesting, then dried in a kiln, then laid to ret in a pond or stream with weighted frames holding them underwater. After retting for three weeks in warm water or five weeks in cold, the stalks were removed and dried for a fortnight or longer, and then again in a kiln for a full day, and then again on racks for the entire winter.[15]

Because most American hemp was produced by the inferior process of dew-retting, rather than water-retting, the resulting product—essentially unsuitable for marine use—was mainly used to make the cheap rope which bound cotton bales. Dew-retted fiber was sufficient for that task, but only a desperate and foolhardy sailor would leave port without water-retted Russian rigging.

tropical merchandise from the West Indies, and furs, to Russia and in trade acquired iron, hemp, and flax—all of which Russia produced in the greatest quantity and the highest quality available in the world at that time. In Russia hemp was treated with such great care and patience that John

The virgin soil of bluegrass country had been unsuitable for grains until the first hemp crop in Kentucky was planted in 1775 to fallow the land for subsequent grain crops. But noting how hemp thrived in bluegrass country, the Kentucky government took a primary interest in hemp for hemp's sake. With an eye to increasing local manufacture, in 1792 Kentucky legislature levied a tax of twenty dollars per ton on hemp imports, which amounted to 3400 tons by 1800. Although Kentucky farmers produced about 6000 tons of fiber in 1810 (when 38 ropewalks were in operation in the state), by 1840 hemp imports had risen to about 5000 tons. The amount dropped to 1500 tons in 1850 after domestic production increased. Before the Civil War, Kentucky farmers employed three slaves per fifty acres to produce about 37,500 pounds of fiber. The "task system" required a slave to produce a daily quota of about one hundred pounds. The slaves received one cent per pound for any amount above the quota, which allowed some of them to earn up to two dollars a day; a few slaves may have been able to buy their freedom in this way. The same system was used in the ropewalks, where a man like William Hayden, who was "acknowl-

edged to be the best spinner in the country," was able to save enough money to buy his freedom in 1824.

In 1841 Congress ordered the U.S. Navy to buy domestic hemp at every opportunity, and in 1843 Congress appropriated fifty thousand dollars to buy American hemp. The navy sent purchasing agents to Kentucky and Missouri to buy domestic, water-retted hemp, but they usually demanded that samples be sent to the Charleston Navy Yard in Massachusetts for inspection before authorizing a purchase. The delay was not worthwhile to growers, and some complained that their fiber had been unfairly rejected by

■■■

Despite the prevalence of hemp cultivation in America, the only documented use of the flowers for intoxication is among slave field hands. Many of the African slave field hands knew about the effects of *dagga* and they would "break up and load their pipes with dried flowering tops of the plants and smoke them,"[16] quietly consuming hemp in peace.

■■■

■■■

Early American Heads of State

Surviving correspondence of the first several presidents of the United States indicates that seven of them smoked cannabis. George Washington allegedly preferred to smoke "the leaves of hemp" rather than to drink alcohol. While campaigning with the Army of the Revolution, General Washington was heard to bemoan that he could not be at home to harvest his hemp crop. James Madison was once heard to say that smoking hemp inspired him to found a new nation on democratic principles.

James Monroe, the fifth U.S. president, was introduced to hashish while he was serving as ambassador to France, and he continued to enjoy the smoke until he was seventy-three years old. When Andrew Jackson, Zachary Taylor, and Franklin Pierce served as military commanders, they each smoked hemp with their soldiers. In one letter to his family, Pierce complained that hemp was "about the only good thing" about the Mexican War.[17]

■■■

Early Kentucky Hemp Fields

James L. Allen paid eloquent tribute to the life of a Kentucky hemp farmer in his 1900 novel *The Reign of Law* revolving around the Bible and hemp husbandry sustained through the seasons and generations:

The Anglo-Saxon farmers had scarce conquered foothold, stronghold, freehold in the Western wilderness before they became sowers of hemp—with remembrance of Virginia, with remembrance of dear ancestral Britain. . . .

The roads of Kentucky, those long limestone turnpikes connecting the towns and villages with the farms— they were early made necessary by the hauling of hemp. For the sake of it slaves were perpetually being trained, hired, bartered; lands perpetually rented and sold; fortunes made or lost . . . .

With the Civil War began the long decline, lasting still. The record stands that throughout the one hundred and twenty-five odd years elapsing from the entrance of the Anglo-Saxon farmers into the wilderness down to the present time, a few counties of Kentucky have furnished army and navy, the entire country, with all but a small part of the native hemp consumed. Little comparatively is cultivated in Kentucky now. The traveller may still see it here and there, self-renewing inexhaustible fields. But the time cannot be far distant when the industry there will have become extinct. Its place in the nation's markets will be still further taken by metals, by other fibres, by finer varieties of the same fibre, by the same variety cultivated in soils less valuable. The history of it in Kentucky will be ended, and, being ended, lost. . . .

Ah! type, too, of our life, which also is earth-sown, earth-rooted; which must struggle upward, be cut down, rotted and broken, ere the separation take place between our dross and our worth—poor perishable shard and immortal fibre. Oh, the mystery, the mystery of that growth from the casting of the soul as a seed into the dark earth, until the time when, led through all natural changes and cleansed of weakness, it is borne from the fields of its nativity for the long service.

From The Reign of Law: A Tale of the Kentucky Hemp Fields, *(London: Macmillan, 1900)*

the inspectors. Accordingly, little Kentucky hemp was bought by the navy. The Kentucky General Assembly appealed to Congress in 1842 to construct a hemp-retting facility as a national security measure. Congress established a rope factory at Memphis in 1852 and equipped it with the best machinery available, but so little southern hemp was forthcoming that the project was abandoned after two years.[18]

Entrepreneurial faith in the hemp industry found new outlets in the mechanical trappings of the industrial revolution. Numerous patents were issued, promising improvements in machinery for the harvesting and preparation of hemp and flax fiber. New hemp breaking and dressing machines promised to cut down on the arduous task of preparing the fiber by hand. G. F. Schaffer of New York patented the Cylinder Flax and Hemp Dresser in 1861, and the following year G. Sanford and J. E. Mallory, also of New York, patented ten improvements for breaking, scutching, cleaning, and dressing hemp.

During the Civil War, the U.S. Congress ordered the North's commissioner of agriculture to make "investigations to test the practicability of cultivating and preparing flax or hemp as a sub-

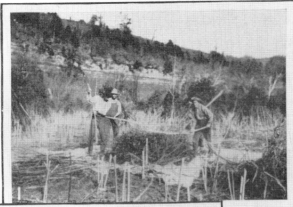

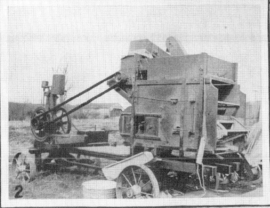

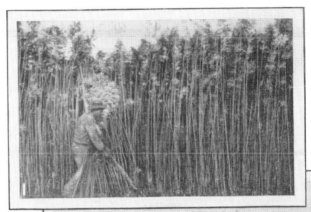

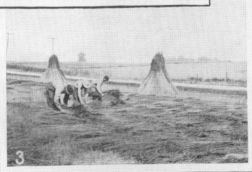

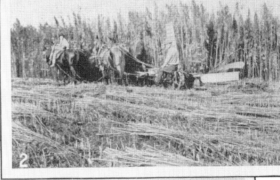

AMERICAN HEMP HARVEST. CUTTING, COLLECTING,
AND RETTING. FROM USDA 1913 YEARBOOK.

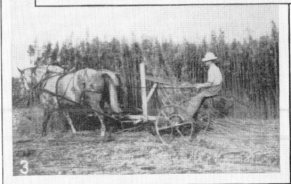

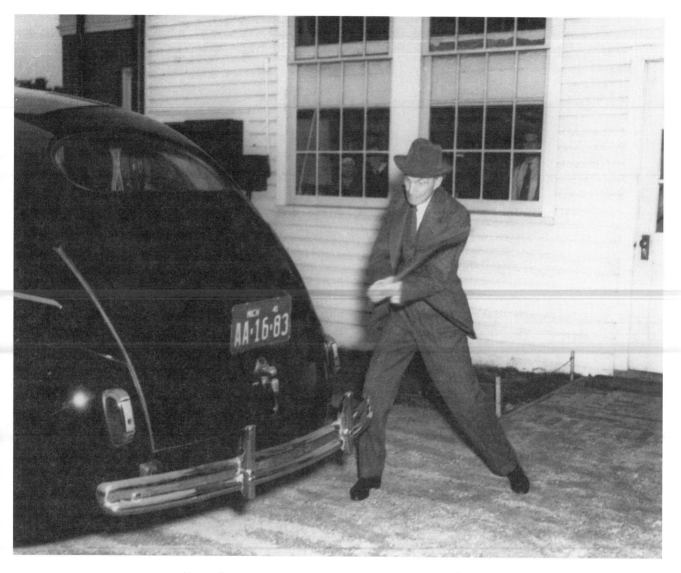

HENRY FORD DEMONSTRATES THE STRENGTH OF HIS CAR "GROWN" FROM A COMBINATION OF HEMP AND OTHER ANNUAL CROPS, AND DESIGNED TO RUN ON HEMP FUEL. PHOTOGRAPH FROM THE COLLECTIONS OF THE HENRY FORD MUSEUM AND GREENFIELD VILLAGE.

stitute for cotton." The war initially caused an increase in the demand for hemp, but the boom was only temporary.[19] After the war, cotton dominated southern agriculture, and cheap imported jute came to replace hemp as the material used to bag cotton. About the same time, wood-pulp paper became widely available and reduced the demand for hemp as a paper-making material. In the aftermath of the Civil War the loss of the slave-labor force and the lack of mechanical harvesters spelled doom for the hemp industry and it never recovered, despite a brief resurgence of hemp cultivation in the 1870s and 1880s.

For a time, hemp was widely grown in Illinois, Nebraska, and California, and the American Flax and Hemp Spinners' and Growers' Association was organized in New York by a dozen manufacturers and merchants in 1882; for several years the society devoted itself largely to lobbying the government to protect the crippled industry. The increasing use of wire cables on ships, and the introduction of steamships and metal hulls, greatly reduced the demand for hemp rope, sails, and caulking.

By the turn of the century the market for hemp was limited to cordage, twine, and thread. But the invention of the mechanical decorticator promised to change that. With sudden easy access to the fiber and cellulose in hemp stalks, inventors raced to create new uses for the prolific plant. Henry Ford, that famous visionary of new trends, foresaw the total

transformation of American industry. Anything currently made from the imported hydrocarbons of the oil molecule could be made from the domestic carbohydrates in hemp. By the 1930s the Ford Motor Company was creating charcoal fuel, creosote, ethyl-acetate, methanol, and other compounds out of hemp at their secret biomass conversion plant at Iron Mountain, Michigan.[20]

Ford envisioned a future where plastics from hemp polymers were the building blocks of almost all products, and where fuel was provided by hemp biomass, and he gave the world a glimpse of that future with his all-organic car.

Mechanical Engineering magazine heralded hemp in its February 1937 issue as "the most profitable and desirable crop that can be grown," and *Popular Mechanics* christened hemp "The New Billion Dollar Crop." Ironically, the article had been written in 1937 but, because of printing schedules, did not appear until 1938. By then passage of the Marihuana Tax Act had rendered the matter moot—the hemp industry was dead.

■ ■ ■

From *Popular Mechanics* magazine, February 1938:

American farmers are promised a new cash crop with an annual value of several hundred million dollars, all because a machine has been invented which solves a problem more than 6,000 years old. It is hemp, a crop which will not compete with other American products. Instead, it will displace imports of raw material and manufactured products produced by underpaid coolie and peasant labor and it will provide thousands of jobs for American workers throughout the land.

The machine which makes this possible is designed for removing the fiber-bearing cortex from the rest of the stalk, making hemp fiber available for use without a prohibitive amount of human labor.

Hemp is a standard fiber of the world. It has great tensile strength and durability. It is used to produce more than 5,000 textile products, ranging from rope to fine laces, and the woody "hurds" remaining after the fiber has been removed contain more than 77% cellulose, and can be used to produce more than 25,000 products, ranging from dynamite to Cellophane. . . .

From the farmers' point of view, hemp is an easy crop to grow and will yield from three to six tons per acre on any land that will grow corn, wheat, or oats. It has a short growing season, so that it can be planted after other crops are in. It can be grown in any state of the union. The long roots penetrate and break the soil to leave it in perfect condition for the next year's crop. The dense shock of leaves, eight to twelve feet above the ground, chokes out weeds. Two successive crops are enough to reclaim land that has been abandoned because of Canadian thistles or quack grass.

Under old methods, hemp was cut and allowed to lie in the fields for weeks until it "retted" enough so the fibers could be pulled off by hand. Retting is simply rotting as a result of dew, rain, and bacterial action. Machines were developed to separate the fibers mechanically after retting was complete, but the cost was high, the loss of fiber great, and the quality of fiber comparatively low. With the new machine, known as a decorticator, hemp is cut with a slightly modified grain binder. It is delivered to the machine where an automatic chain conveyor feeds it to the breaking arms at the rate of two or three tons per hour. The hurds are broken into fine pieces which drop into the hopper, from where they are delivered by blower to a baler or to a truck or freight car for loose shipment. The fiber comes from the other end of the machine, ready for baling.

From this point on almost anything can happen. The raw fiber can be used to produce strong twine or rope, woven into burlap, used for carpet warp or linoleum backing or it may be bleached and refined, with resinous by-products of high commercial value. It can, in fact, be used to replace the foreign fibers which now flood our markets.

Thousands of tons of hemp hurds are used every year by one large powder company for the manufacture of dynamite and TNT. A large paper company, which has been paying more than a million dollars a year in duties on foreign-made cigarette papers, now is manufacturing these papers from American hemp grown in Minnesota. A new factory in Illinois is producing fine bond papers from hemp. The natural materials in hemp make it an economical source of pulp for any grade of paper manufactured, and the high percentage of alpha-cellulose promises an unlimited supply of raw material for the thousands of cellulose products our chemists have developed.

It is generally believed that all linen is produced from flax. Actually, the majority comes from hemp—authorities estimate that more than half of our imported linen fabrics are manufactured from hemp fiber. Another misconception is that burlap is made from hemp. Actually, its source is usually jute, and practically all of the burlap we use is woven by laborers in India who receive only four cents a day. Binder twine is usually made from sisal which comes from Yucatan and East Africa.

All of these products, now imported, can be produced from home-grown hemp. Fish nets, bow strings, canvas, strong rope, overalls, damask tablecloths, fine linen garments, towels, bed linen and thousands of other everyday items can be grown on American farms. Our imports of foreign fabrics and fibers average about $200,000,000 per year; in raw fibers alone we imported over $50,000,000 in the first six months of 1937. All this income can be made available for Americans.

The paper industry offers even greater possibilities. As an industry it amounts to over $1,000,000,000 a year, and of that 80% is imported. But hemp will produce every grade of paper, and government figures estimate that 10,000 acres devoted to hemp will produce as much paper as 40,000 acres of average pulp land.

■■■

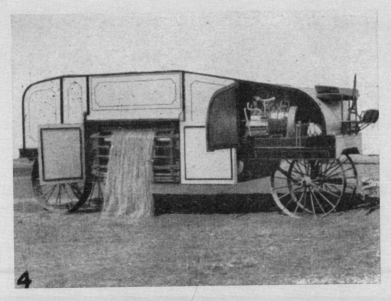

A DECORTICATOR USED IN 1913. PHOTOGRAPH FROM USDA 1913 YEARBOOK.

6

MARIJUANA
MADNESS

Cannabism in
America

I n the second half of the nineteenth century, thousands of Americans rediscovered the ancient pleasures of cannabis in the form of hashish and ganja imported from India and Egypt. The American diplomat

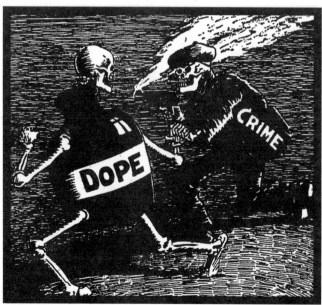

HEARST NEWSPAPER ILLUSTRATION. HAND-RETOUCHED BY RODDY HEADING.

Bayard Taylor wrote accounts of his experience with hashish for magazines as well as in his memoir *Land of the Saracens*. In one chapter, "The Vision of Hashish," Taylor asserts that it revealed to him "deeps of rapture and suffering which my natural faculties never could have sounded." As a youth, Fitz Hugh Ludlow, the son of an abolitionist minister, read Thomas de Quincey's *Confessions of an English Opium-Eater,* and in 1854, when he was eighteen, Ludlow also read Bayard Taylor's descriptions of his experience with hashish while in Damascus.

Taylor's writing moved Ludlow "powerfully to curiosity and admiration." After two years of experimentation with hashish, Ludlow quit his trials. He describes the experience in his 1854 memoir, *The Hasheesh Eater*.[1] Ludlow's account captured the attention and imagination of many curious people, some of whom began to experiment with hashish firsthand. Eighteen-year-old John Hay—who would later become an aide to President Abraham Lincoln—tried it and told a friend it was "a marvelous stimulant to the imagination." In later days this former presidential aide and secretary of state reminisced about when he "used to eat Hasheesh and dream dreams . . . in a mystical Eden." Without fear of public censure, others felt free to follow the lead of an adventurous few once the herb became more widely available.

Far from being considered a dangerous and potentially disruptive "drug," hashish was marketed as a "candy" and consumed in the spirit of recreation and relaxation. The Gunjah Wallah Company of New York began marketing "hasheesh candy" in the 1860s, advertising: "The Arabian Gunje of Enchantment confectionized—A most pleasurable and harmless stimulant." The company even claimed that the

sweet would cure "Nervousness, Weakness, Melancholy," and would inspire "all classes with new life and energy." The popular product was marketed for forty years, a testament to the social acceptance of cannabis. Other early appearances of cannabis included the 1876 Centennial Exposition in Philadelphia. This event featured a fashionable Turkish Hashish Exposition that pulled in crowds of people who seemed to prefer smoking rather than eating hashish: the effects were felt immediately, and the smokers could control their intake puff by puff, stopping when satisfied.[2]

Cannabis was considered to be an aphrodisiac, and experts recommended it as such in several late nineteenth-century marriage manuals. In his *Marriage Guide* of 1850, "doctor" Frederick Hollick of Philadelphia advised troubled couples to use hashish to stimulate their libido, and he manufactured a preparation that he advertised for this purpose. If Hollick's love potion didn't lead to amorous reconciliation, at least it didn't contribute to violence. Prevailing popular opinion blamed domestic disharmony on alcohol, and in the 1890s several women's temperance societies actually recommended the recreational use of hashish rather than alcohol,

Cannabis and romance are linked in Louisa May Alcott's "Perilous Play," a short story published anonymously in Frank Leslie's *Chimney Corner* on 13 February 1869. The tale relates the adventures of a party of bored young socialites who indulge in some hashish candy. Two of the characters become lost together on a sailboat, but they survive and find true love. The story ends with their safe return to the party during which the heroine pleads:

"Oh, Mr. Done, screen me from their eyes and questions as much as you can! I'm so worn out and nervous, I shall betray myself. You will help me?" And she turned to him with a confiding look, strangely at variance with her usual calm self-possession.

"I'll shield you with my life, if you will tell me why you took the hashish," he said, bent on knowing his fate.

"I hoped it would make me soft and lovable, like other women. I'm tired of being a lonely statue," she faltered, as if the truth was wrung from her by a power stronger than her will.

"And I took it to gain courage to tell my love. Rose, we have been near death together; let us share life together, and neither of us be any more lonely or afraid?"

He stretched his hand to her with his heart in his face, and she gave him hers with a look of tender submission, as he said ardently, "Heaven bless hashish, if its dreams end like this!"[3]

because they believed that liquor led to wife-beating while hashish did not.

Despite such random entrées into popular culture, hashish remained obscure—illicit but not illegal—in the late Victorian era. Beginning in the 1800s, "hasheesh houses" by the hundreds catered to wealthy sophisticates in New York and other major cities—but secrecy was the rule. The Pure Food and Drug Act of 1906 was the first federal law directly to concern cannabis, but even this law merely stated that any quantity of the substance (and several others such as alcohol, opium, cocaine and chloral hydrate) had to be clearly stated on the label of any food or drug sold to the public.

Early Drug Prohibition

Social reformers tried to include cannabis in the proscriptions of the Harrison Act of 1914, but the pharmaceutical industry successfully opposed its inclusion since it was an ingredient of corn plasters and several other medicaments and was widely used in veterinary medicine. The Harrison Act required importers, producers, and dealers in opium and coca prod-

ucts to register and pay an occupational tax. The registered parties had to file detailed reports of their drug transactions, each of which was recorded on an official order form. The awkward procedures were designed to be unworkable in practice, indirectly discouraging traffic in opiates and cocaine. In the 1919 Supreme Court decision *United States v. Doremus,* which upheld the Harrison Act by a five-to-four vote, the dissenting judges argued that "the statute was a mere attempt by Congress to exert a power not delegated, that is, the reserved police power of the States." Congress used this obtuse approach in regulating drugs by taxation because, as the Supreme Court confirmed in its 1925 decision *Linder v. United States*, "direct control of medical practice in the states is beyond the power of the Federal Government," according to the Tenth Amendment.[4]

Early legislation against narcotics consisted largely of ad hoc local attempts to "do something" about a problem that arguably did not exist. Fear of cannabis seemed more to reflect society's fear of the unfettered human mind; marijuana was aptly described in a jazz song of the era as "the stuff that dreams are made of . . . the thing that white folks are afraid of." The Louisiana legislature in 1911 thus prohibited pharmacists from refilling prescriptions which contained cannabis, opium, or cocaine, among other drugs. The city of El Paso, Texas, passed an ordinance to ban the sale and possession of marijuana in 1914; that same year the city of New York added "*Cannabis indica,* which is the Indian hemp from which the East Indian drug called hashish is manufactured," to its list of proscribed drugs. The *New York Times* reported on this amendment of the sanitary code on 30 July 1914 and editorialized that cannabis was a narcotic having "practically the same effect as morphine and cocaine. . . . The inclusion of *Cannabis indica* among the drugs to be sold only on prescription is only common sense. Devotees of hashish are now hardly numerous enough here to count, but they are likely to increase as other narcotics become harder to obtain."

By 1915 several New England states, along with California, Utah, and Wyoming, had passed laws against cannabis in anticipation of possible problems. Texas passed a law against cannabis in 1919, and Iowa, Nevada, Oregon, Washington, Arkansas, and Nebraska followed suit in 1923. Meanwhile the federal prohibition against alcohol—with the passage of the Eighteenth Amendment in 1919,

and its enforcement legislature, the Volstead Act of 1920—had made alcohol more costly, difficult to acquire, and dangerous to use. The market for cannabis, which was federally uncontrolled, increased to meet the intractable human demand for intoxicants.

Racist Propaganda, Conspiracy, and Cannabis

When a clique of New Orleans city officials blamed marijuana for creating a crime wave in 1926 the issue was finally transmuted into a mountain of political hay that reached Washington, D.C. The *New Orleans Item* and the *Morning Tribune* newspapers ran sensationalized reports focusing on marijuana's use by "children," who were in fact street-wise youths and anything but innocent victims: "School children [could buy marijuana cigarettes] almost as readily as sandwiches. Their cost was two for a quarter. The children solved the problem of cost by pooling pennies among the members of a group and then passing the cigarettes from one to another, all the puffs being carefully counted." The New Orleans coroner offered a pseudoscientific

The term *marijuana*, popularized by the Hearst newspapers in the 1930s, is not, as people sometimes assume, the Spanish word for cannabis. *Cáñamo* is. But the obscure slang term *marijuana* was used to alarm the public and kept experts from comparing the outlandish claims regarding the "Mexican drug" with the known qualities of hemp.[5]

explanation for the supposed link between crime and marijuana; the substance, he maintained, "stimulates the cortical cerebral centers and inhibits the controlling subcortical centers of [the] mechanism which is responsible for . . . bolstering up their courage and the various phenomena which will eventually . . . lead them into the most crime-producing individuals that we have."

Soon afterward, in 1927, the Louisiana legislature passed a law imposing a maximum penalty of six months in jail or a $500 fine for the possession or sale of marijuana. Highly publicized roundups resulted in "a wholesale arrest of more than 150 persons." Approximately one hundred underworld

dives, soft-drink establishments, night clubs, grocery stores, and private homes were searched in the police raids. Addicts, hardened criminals, gangsters, prostitutes, sailors of all nationalities, bootleggers, even boys and girls were rounded up in an early attempt to wage a "war" on cannabis.

The misdirected effort at prohibition in Louisiana was utterly futile. The state's narcotics officer declared in 1936 that "60 percent of the crimes committed in New Orleans were by marihuana users. . . . Practically every negro in the city can give a recognizable description of the drug's effects. . . . Cigarettes are hard to get and are selling at 30 to 40 cents apiece, which is a relatively high price and a particularly good indication of the effectiveness of the present control." In other words, a decade of law enforcement had merely doubled the price of cannabis cigarettes without reducing consumption, which had become endemic.

The negative propaganda emanating from Louisiana had an inordinate influence on the national perception of cannabis. Since 1915 public perception of hemp had been strongly influenced by newspaper and magazine articles that ascribed every evil to the influence of marijuana, just as

The crusading demagogue Dr. A. E. Fossier resuscitated the myth of the *hashishin* Assassins in the *New Orleans Medical and Surgical Journal* in 1931.

The underworld was quick to realize that marihuana was an ideal drug to quickly cut off the inhibition, especially in the light of inadequate personality . . . Under the influence of cannabis indica, these human derelicts are quickly subjugated by the will of the master mind. The moral principles or training initiated in the mind from in-fancy may deter from committing willful theft, murder or rape, but this inhibition from crime may be destroyed by the addiction to marihuana. . . . The debasing and baneful influence of hashish and opium is not restricted to individuals but has manifested itself in nations and races as well. The dominant race and most enlightened countries are alcoholic, whilst the races and nations addicted to hemp and opium, some of which once attained to heights of culture and civilization, have deteriorated both mentally and physically.[6]

opium and cocaine had been demonized and vilified years before. But now a spate of unsubstantiated accounts in popular magazines featured such titles as "Marijuana: Assassin of Youth" (in *American Magazine*), "Sex Crazing Drug Menace" (in *Physical Culture*), and "Youth Gone Loco" (in *Christian Century*). Among the many dreadful effects attributed to "the menace of marihuana" in the *International Medical Digest,* was that "a boy and a girl . . . had lost their senses so completely after smoking marijuana [they] eloped and were married."[7]

An unqualified article linking marijuana, crime, and insanity appeared in the *Journal of Criminal Law and Criminology* in 1932, and was often cited thereafter as a definitive study. The authors, L. E. Bowery, a policeman from Wichita, Kansas, and M. A. Hayes asserted that the marijuana user is capable of

> great feats of strength and endurance, during which no fatigue is felt. . . . Sexual desires are stimulated and may lead to unnatural acts, such as indecent exposure and rape. . . . [Use of marijuana] ends in the destruction of brain tissues and nerve centers, and does irreparable damage. If continued, the inevitable result is insanity,

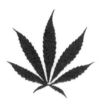

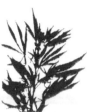

ANTI-MARIJUANA PROPAGANDA CIRCULATED BY THE DIVISION OF NARCOTIC ENFORCEMENT.

which those familiar with it describe as absolutely incurable, and, without exception ending in death.

Although moral entrepreneurs were wont to claim that marijuana was a heinous, seductive narcotic that caused insanity and crime, *Cannabis sativa* was suppressed in America for reasons that had as much to do with racism and economics as with morality. A free-for-all association linking "marijuana madness" with Mexicans, African Americans, jazz music, sex, and violence had been embraced by American propagandists, whose fears and fantasies were indulged by the media. "Keep America

---

Between 1943 and 1948 Harry Anslinger's Federal Bureau of Narcotics maintained constant surveillance and extensive files on many musicians, singers, actors, and comedians, including such greats as Louis Armstrong, Count Basie, Milton Berle, Les Brown, Cab Calloway, Jimmy Dorsey, Duke Ellington, Dizzy Gillespie, Jackie Gleason, Lionel Hampton, Andre Kostelanetz, Kate Smith, and the entire NBC Orchestra. Anslinger's files weren't arbitrary: Armstrong had been busted for possession of marijuana in 1931 and received a six-month suspended sentence after spending ten days in jail. The great jazz drummer Gene Krupa served time in San Quentin prison for possession of marijuana and for involving a minor. Harry Anslinger planned to orchestrate a nationwide roundup of all his suspects, but his superior in the Treasury Department, Assistant Secretary Foley, cancelled it with a memo: "Mr. Foley disapproves!"[8]

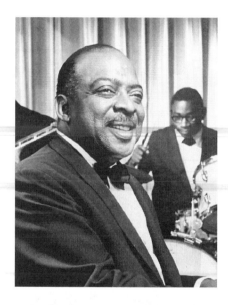

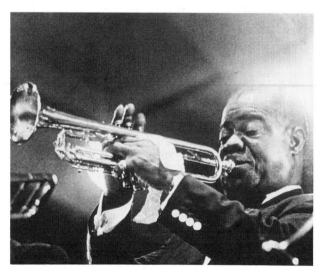

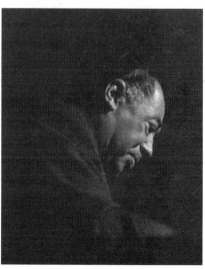

TOP: COUNT BASIE; BOTTOM: DUKE ELLINGTON; LEFT: LOUIS ARMSTRONG.

American" framed the scapegoating of racial minorities and waves of new immigrants, who were projected as a threat to the nation's morality in sensational front-page stories that found their epitome in the yellow journalism of William Randolph Hearst. Hearst hated minorities, and he used his chain of papers to aggravate racial tensions at every opportunity. Hearst papers were known to claim that cocaine caused negroes to rape white women—until cocaine went out of vogue, at which point marijuana became responsible for negroes raping white women.[9]

Hearst especially hated Mexicans. Hearst papers portrayed Mexicans as lazy, degenerate, and violent, and as marijuana smokers and job stealers. The real motive behind this prejudice may well have been that Hearst had lost 800,000 acres of prime timberland to the rebel army of Pancho Villa, suggesting that Hearst's racism was fueled by Mexican threat to his empire.

Hemp activist Jack Herer, author of the 1994 book *The Emperor Wears No Clothes*, argues convincingly that cannabis was suppressed in America not just for "moral" reasons but for economic ones. Hemp products threatened certain vested financial and industrial interests, which conspired to destroy the industry by supporting the zealous moral reformers who sought its prohibition at the federal level. The petrochemical and pulp-paper industries in particular stood to lose billions of dollars if the commercial potential of hemp was fully realized. Herer names Hearst and Du Pont as two of the interests most responsible for orchestrating the demise of hemp manufacture. In the 1920s the Du Pont company developed and patented fuel additives such as tetraethyl lead, as well as the sulfate and sulfite processes for manufacture of pulp paper and numerous new synthetic products such as nylon, cellophane, and other plastics. At the same time, other companies were developing synthetic products from renewable biomass resources—especially hemp. The hemp decorticator promised to eliminate much of the need for wood-pulp paper, thus threatening to drastically reduce the value of the vast timberlands still owned by Hearst. Ford and other companies were already promising to make every product from cannabis carbohydrates that was currently being made from petroleum hydrocarbons. In response, from 1935 to 1937, Du Pont lobbied the chief counsel of the Treasury Department, Herman Oliphant, for the prohibition of

---

■■■

Marijuana was sometimes called Mezzrole after Milton "Mezz" Mezzrow, a white musician who called himself a "voluntary Negro." Mezzrow moved from Chicago to Harlem in 1929 and began selling high-grade marijuana cigarettes on the streets. In his autobiography *Really the Blues* he said, "Overnight I was the most popular man in Harlem."[10]

New Orleans jazz master Louis Armstrong once characterized the criminalization of marijuana as one might a love affair gone sour: "One reason we appreciated pot was the warmth it always brought forth. . . . Mary Warner, honey, you sure was good and I enjoyed you heap much. But the price got a little too high to pay, law wise. At first you was a misdemeanor. But as the years rolled by you lost your 'misde' and got meaner and meaner."

■■■

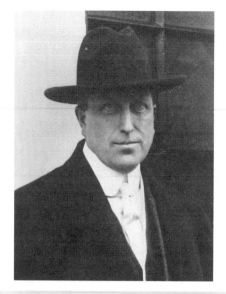

WILLIAM RANDOLPH HEARST, OWNER OF A MAJOR NEWSPAPER CHAIN, INTRODUCED THE TERM MARIHUANA TO THE AMERICAN PUBLIC. HE OWNED VAST TIMBER HOLDINGS WHICH FED THE PAPER INDUSTRY, WHICH USED CHEMICALS DEVELOPED BY DU PONT.

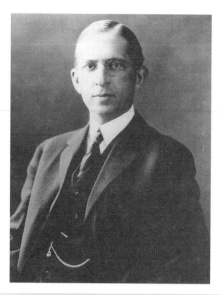

LAMMONT DU PONT, PRESIDENT OF THE DU PONT COMPANY, DOMINATED THE PETROCHEMICAL MARKET, MANUFAC-TURING PLASTICS, PAINTS, AND OTHER PRODUCTS FROM FOSSIL FUELS.

cannabis, assuring him that Du Pont's synthetic petrochemicals (such as urethane) could replace hemp-seed oil in the marketplace.[11]

Some large pharmaceutical companies also stood to gain by the illegalization of cannabis, since their synthetic patented prescription tranquilizers (such as barbiturates) would find room in the void left by prohibition of this natural relaxant. At the same time, some companies were distributing tons of marijuana in Texas and the southwest, where it was sold over the counter in one-ounce packages, in tinctures, and by mail order. In El Paso, Texas, druggists were interviewed for a report to the USDA to determine whether Mexican "loco-weed" was a problem requiring federal intervention. The responses of the pharmacists dutifully reflected—and perpetuated—racist propaganda in association with marijuana. With no pretense to objectivity, the government report asserts that marijuana was purchased by Mexicans "of low birth" for recreation and for medi-cinal purposes including the treatment of venereal disease; other purchasers included Negroes, chauffeurs, and a low class of whites such as those addicted to the use of habit-forming drugs and hangers-on of the underworld.[12] With propaganda and lobbying,

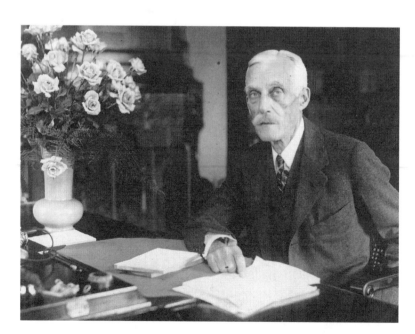

ANDREW MELLON, SECRETARY OF THE TREASURY AND OWNER OF GULF OIL, WAS THE RICHEST MAN IN AMERICA. HE LENT DU PONT MONEY TO PURCHASE GENERAL MOTORS, AND PUSHED LEGISLATION THROUGH CONGRESS GIVING TAX BREAKS TO OIL COMPANIES.

Du Pont, Hearst, and their associates threw their efforts into crushing the competition posed by hemp, and they succeeded.

Harry Anslinger and The Uniform Narcotics Act

On 30 October 1929 a Texas senator introduced a bill (S. 2075) to amend the Narcotics Drugs Import and Export Act of 1922 to include cannabis. Other congressmen urged the Bureau of Prohibition to add a tax on cannabis to the Harrison Act. The Bureau of Prohibition opposed both proposals because hemp was a domestic crop. As such, it could not be controlled by federal legislature unless it involved interstate or international commerce, according to the constitutional separation of state and federal powers. Therefore, the Bureau of Prohibition promoted a Uniform Narcotic Act, which made the states responsible for enforcing the law. The bureau had already tried to promote international control of cannabis by the League of Nations, but the American proposals were rebuffed at the Second Geneva Opium Conference in 1925.[13]

In preparing the bureau's position paper on S. 2075 (which later died in committee), secretary Harry Anslinger of the Federal Narcotics Control Board asked the American Medical Association and the American Drug Manufacturers' Association several questions about the use of cannabis in medicine. The AMA resented any increase in governmental control of physicians and pharmacists, and Dr. William C. Woodward, director of the AMA's Bureau of Legal Medicine, wrote a caustic reply to Anslinger advising him to direct his questions to the appropriate government agencies. Dr. Woodward had worked with the AMA since 1922 to test the feasibility of including cannabis in the Uniform Act, and he had conducted an independent survey to gather pharmacists' opinions on the matter. All but one respondent had refuted the popular view that cannabis was addictive or even "habit-forming," and none knew of any abuse of its pharmaceutical preparations.

The Federal Bureau of Narcotics (FBN) was established on 12 August 1930 under the aegis of the Treasury Department with Harry J. Anslinger appointed as the FBN's first commissioner. In the first few years after its inception, Anslinger's FBN minimized the marijuana issue and argued that the individual states should control the problem. The Bureau of Narcotics was hard-pressed to survive in the depression's weakened economy, and initially it limited its efforts to enforcing the Harrison Act against opium and cocaine and promoting the passage of the Uniform Act. But eventually Anslinger's attention turned toward cannabis. Did Anslinger generate the issue as a way to ensure the survival of the tiny FBN? We don't know. What we do know is that Anslinger was nephew-in-law to Secretary of the Treasury Andrew Mellon, a banker who was financing the growing petrochemical dynasty of the Du Ponts. Mellon had designed Anslinger's position personally.[14]

Immediately after becoming FBN commissioner—a position he held until ousted by John F. Kennedy in 1962—Harry Anslinger tried to get his agency involved in the drafting process of "the AMA Bill," the Uniform Narcotic Drug Act. When a conference was held on 15 September 1932 representatives of all the interested parties were there: a judicial subcommittee, the Department of State, the American Medical Association, the Public Health Service, members of the pharmaceutical and health professions and industries, and the Federal Bureau of Narcotics. The final draft of the AMA Bill was agreed upon for presentation to the National Conference of State Commissioners the next month. The industrial interests considered the prohibition of cannabis to be untenable, however, and the counsel of the National Association of Retail Druggists, E. Brookmeyer, said so in no uncertain terms: "Strike the cannabis section. . . . The abuse complained of is altogether local." Section 12 on cannabis was eliminated, and it was left to the conference of state commissioners to decide whether it should be included in the act. The National Conference of Commissioners on the Uniform Drug Act met on 8 October 1932, and adopted the fifth draft of the bill with a vote of twenty-six to three. However, the optional provision for cannabis defined the plant as a "narcotic" in all states, technically equivalent to opium, and subject to the same draconian penalties.

Anslinger immediately directed his three hundred FBN agents to assist the sponsors of the Uniform Act both by lobbying the state legislatures to enact the proposed law and by conducting a relentless publicity campaign to enlist public support. Objections to the act nonetheless proved formidable. The potential costs of enforcement and the attendant paperwork were excessive, and there was considerable misunderstanding of the Uniform Act's requirements, technicalities, and exemptions. Despite these obstacles, the fight to pass the act was bringing marijuana out of obscurity and into the public eye. Now that a "sympathetic public interest, helpful to the administration of the narcotic laws" had been aroused, Harry Anslinger would make sure it would be maintained.

Nonetheless, by 1935 the Uniform Act had been passed by only ten states. Frustrated in his attempts to convince legislators and citizens of the need for the unglamorous new law, Anslinger decided to intensify his propaganda campaign to arouse public fear of the "marihuana menace," thus pressuring legislators to take action. As the FBN's "educational campaign to describe the weed and tell of its horrible effects" reached a peak of frenzy, no statement was too ridiculous to be said and printed. "If the hideous monster Frankenstein came face to face with the monster Marihuana, he would drop dead of fright," hyperbolized Anslinger, in William Randolph Hearst's *Washington Herald* of 12 April 1937. Hearst provided many of the fantastic stories that Anslinger used to en-

hance the articles he authored. The infamous article "Marihuana: Assassin of Youth," which appeared in *American Magazine* in July of 1937, began with a grisly scene that never occurred:

> The sprawled body of a young girl lay crushed on the sidewalk the other day after a plunge from the fifth story of a Chicago apartment house. Everyone called it suicide but actually it was murder. The killer was a narcotic known to America as marihuana, and history as hashish. It is a narcotic used in the form of cigarettes, comparatively new to the United States and as dangerous as a coiled rattlesnake.[15]

The FBN received dozens of letters addressed to Anslinger. "Your article was the first time I ever heard of marihuana," wrote one citizen. In the two years after publication of the story, it was excerpted with credit to Anslinger in four of at least sixteen other magazine articles printed about cannabis during that period. Few if any of Anslinger's stories about murder and rape committed under the influence of marijuana were in fact true.[16] But in his 1961 book *The Murderers* Anslinger boasts, "I believe we did a thorough job, for the public was

> ■■■
>
> "Marijuana-smoking at women's bridge parties has become frequent, the parties usually ending up in wild carousals, sometimes with men joining the orgies."
>
> *Union Signal,* October 1934
>
> ■■■

153

alerted, and the laws to protect them were passed, both nationally and at the state level." Although his sensational stories were never verifiable, his claim that the FBN cleaned up most of the country's wild-growing marijuana seems to be true. "There were still some WPA gangs working in those days and we put them to good use," he writes. As Anslinger describes it:

Just outside the nation's capital, for some sixty miles along the Potomac River, on both banks, marijuana was growing in profusion; it had been planted there originally by early settlers who made their own hemp and cloth. The workers cleaned out tremendous river bank crops, destroying plants, seeds and roots. All through the Midwest also, WPA workers were used for this cleanup job. The wild hemp was rooted out of America.[17]

The Marihuana Tax Act

A letter to the Federal Bureau of Narcotics from the editor of the Alamosa, Colorado *Daily Courier* reflects the fear, ignorance, and racism surrounding public concern over marijuana by 1936:

Can you enlarge your Department to deal with marijuana? . . . I wish you could see what a small cigarette can do to one of our degenerate Spanish-speaking residents. That's why our problem is so great: the greatest percentage of our population is composed of Spanish-speaking persons, most of whom are low mentally, because of social and racial conditions.

While marijuana has figured in the greatest number of crimes in the past few years, officials fear it, not for what it has done, but for what it is capable of doing. They want to check it before an outbreak does occur.

Local law-enforcement agencies also appealed to their state governors, who pressured Henry Morgenthau, Jr., the secretary of the treasury, to take action. He in turn assigned the Treasury's general counsel, Herman Oliphant, to draft appropriate legislation; however, Oliphant was unable to find a suitable constitutional basis for the prohibition of hemp. Eventually, he chose to use the models of the Harrison Narcotics Act and the National Firearms Act, which imposed a prohibitive "transfer tax" on the sale of machine guns. Knowing the Firearms Act had been declared constitutional by the Supreme Court in March

1937, Oliphant decided that a transfer tax might be applied successfully to marijuana. FBN Commissioner Anslinger at first thought the idea was absurd and expressed doubt that Congress would accept it. Many honest Americans, after all, still made their living with hemp. In January 1936 he met with several experts in New York to draft a bill, but had to conclude in a confidential report to Stephen Gibbons, the assistant secretary of the treasury, that "under the taxing power and regulation of interstate commerce it would be almost hopeless to expect any kind of adequate control." He suggested instead that an international treaty be made to control the alleged problem.

Anslinger and Stuart Fuller of the State Department presented the idea of a treaty to control cannabis at the Conference for the Suppression of Illicit Traffic in Dangerous Drugs, held in Geneva in June 1936, but their proposal was rejected by the twenty-six other nations at the conference. Oliphant and Anslinger continued to prepare the Marihuana Tax Act in secret for presentation to Congress. They gathered scientific and medical opinions, ignoring any information that did not concur with their bias against hemp. The Treasury Department was not inter-

ested in educated opinions. To the contrary, Treasury attorney S. G. Tipton asked Commissioner Anslinger: "Have you lots of cases on this? Horror stories—that's what we want." Tipton got the stories, and presented them with their case for HR 6385 to the six-member House Ways and Means Committee in April 1937.

The House Ways and Means Committee was chosen because it is the only committee that sends bills directly to the House of Representatives without debate from other committees. Committee chairman Robert L. Doughton of North Carolina happened to be an ally of the Du Pont dynasty, which was poised to reap enormous profits from the suppression of hemp. The bill was voted on without a roll call and passed on to the Senate Committee on Finance, which was controlled by Prentice Brown of Michigan, another ally of Du Pont.[18]

Chairman Doughton called the Ways and Means Committee meeting to order on 11 May 1937, "for the purpose of considering HR 6385 . . . a bill to impose an occupational excise tax upon certain dealers in marijuana, to impose a transfer tax upon certain dealings in marijuana, and to safeguard the revenue therefrom by registry and recording."[19]

■ ■ ■

Alarmist hyperbole regarding the supposed dangers of cannabis ingestion is nothing new. The tenth-century Ibn Wahshiyah wrote of the potent cannabis preparation hashish in his book *On Poisons*, and claimed that the "odor" is deadly:

If it reaches the nose, a violent tickle occurs in the nose, then in the face. The face and eyes are affected by an extreme and intense burning; one does not see anything and cannot say what one wishes. One swoons, then recovers, then swoons again and recovers again. One goes on this way until he dies.

■ ■ ■

Clinton Hester, the Treasury Department's assistant general counsel, claimed that

The purpose of HR 6385 is to employ the federal taxing power not only to raise revenue from the marihuana traffic, but also to discourage the current and widespread undesirable use of marihuana by smokers and drug addicts and thus drive the traffic into channels where the plant will be put to valuable industrial, medical and scientific uses. . . . Although the $100 transfer tax in this bill is intended to be prohibitive, as is the $200 transfer tax in the National Firearms Act, it is submitted that it is constitutional as a revenue measure.

Harry Anslinger testified and surpassed his own reputation for rhetoric, arguing:

This traffic in marijuana is increasing to such an extent that it has become the cause for the greatest national concern. In medical schools the physician-to-be is taught that without opium medicine would be like a one-armed man. That is true, because you cannot get along without opium. But here is a drug that is not like opium. Opium has all the good of Dr. Jekyll and all the evil of Mr. Hyde. This drug is entirely the monster Hyde, the harmful effect of which cannot be measured.

Others testifying at the meeting brought more positive information to the committee's attention, including a manufacturer of pigeon feed, who was clear in his conviction that there was no acceptable substitute for hemp seed in the production of well-bred squabs. Pigeons need to consume hemp oil, he explained: it brought back their feathers but did not turn them into marijuana addicts. The committee heard more pertinent testimony from Dr. William C. Woodward, legislative counsel for the AMA, who opined that the proposed law was contrived. He criticized every aspect of the bill, beginning with the selective and deficient nature of the testimony offered by the FBN.

The Bureau of the Public Health Service has also a division of pharmacology. If you desire evidence as to the pharmacology of *Cannabis,* that obviously is the place where you can get direct and primary evidence, rather than the indirect hearsay evidence. . . . There is nothing in the medical use of *Cannabis* that has any relation to *Cannabis* addiction. I use the word *"Cannabis"* in preference to *"marijuana,"* because cannabis is the correct term for describing the plant and its products. The term "marijuana" is a mongrel word that has crept into this country over the Mexican border and has no general meaning, except as it relates to the use of *Cannabis* preparations for smoking.

Woodward's doubts about the bill's practicability, and his insistence that marijuana was not a drug that had anything to do with medicine or the AMA left the committee in a fit of pique. Cutting off Woodward's answers, the committee nonetheless pressed with questions: Why didn't Woodward write his own legislation if he didn't like this bill? Was Woodward trying to throw obstacles in the government's way? Was Woodward resentful because no one consulted him about the bill? "Without legislative control . . . we would have no civilization whatever," huffed committee chairman Doughton, taking the last word and calling the committee to recess.

Ralph Loziers, the general counsel of the National Oil Seed Institute, was another of the few dissenting voices at the House hearings. Loziers argued that the bill calling for a prohibitive tax on the sale of cannabis was too

all-inclusive, and he rose to defend importation of hemp seed, pointing out that "[the] seed of the *Cannabis sativa* L. is used in all the Oriental nations and also in a part of Russia as food. It is grown in their fields and used as oatmeal. Millions of people every day are using hemp seed in the Orient as food. They have been doing that for many generations, especially in periods of famine."

The *Journal of the American Medical Association* published a strong editorial in belated response against the proposed federal law in its 1 May 1937 issue. Pharmacists and physicians rarely needed to dispense cannabis, said the journal,

but they must nevertheless be prepared to dispense it when a call does come, so they will have to pay the tax. . . . All this will be in the end paid for by the patient and thus will go to swell the cost of sickness. Thus the sick and injured must contribute toward efforts to suppress a habit that has little or no relation to the use of cannabis for medical purposes.

The bill was presented to the full House on 14 June 1937. Only four representatives asked for an explanation of the bill and in response a member of the Ways

Harry Anslinger seemed to believe his own rhetoric about marijuana's fearful potency. In the midst of the crackdown on marijuana-smoking jazz musicians, Anslinger was appointed in 1942 to a top-secret committee assigned to discover a "truth serum" for the Office of Strategic Services to use on suspected spies. The first substance he suggested was pure cannabis resin! Use of cannabis was discontinued after fifteen months because it proved to be unreliable; the subjects would either laugh or get paranoid, and then get hungry. Futher complicating things was the discovery that agents were withholding the resin from suspected spies and instead using it themselves.[20]

An exerpt from the House "debate" on the Marihuana Tax Act raises questions about not only the bill in question but the entire process of legislation.

Congressman Snell: "Is this a matter we should bring up at this late hour of the afternoon? I do not know anything about the bill. It may be all right and it may be that everyone is for it, but as a general principle, I am against bringing up any important legislation, and I suppose this is important, since it comes from the Ways and Means Committee, at this late hour of the day."

Congressman Rayburn: "Mr. Speaker, if the gentleman will yield, I may say that the gentleman from North Carolina has stated to me that this bill has a unanimous report from the committee and that there is no controversy about it."

Mr. Snell: "What is the bill?"

Mr. Rayburn: "It has something to do with something that is called marihuana. I believe it is a narcotic of some kind."[21]

■■■

and Means Committee offered an account of criminal acts allegedly connected to the use of marijuana. The act passed the House without controversy and was forwarded to the Senate Committee on Finance. The subcommittee hearing was held on July 12 of that year.

As the first witness, Harry Anslinger read several more horror stories for the record, attempting to discredit cannabis's medical utility and to deny the law's impact on the legitimate hemp industry. But Matt Rens, founder of the Rens Hemp Company of Brandon, Wisconsin, entered into the record a statement that interpreted

the bill in relation to legitimate hemp producers and suggested some changes. Rens asked that the five-dollar fee be reduced to one dollar for the sake of the many small farmers who produced only a few acres or less of hemp for seed. The superintendent of the AmHempCo Corporation of Danville, Illinois, appeared as a witness for the industry and also complained about the $5 tax. Although the capacity of his factory was fifteen thousand acres, he said, the company had only seven thousand acres planted.

We have to contract our seed from growers [whose] acreage runs anywhere from a quarter of an acre up, and we have no objection to the bill. In fact, any attempt to prevent the passage of a bill to protect the narcotic traffic would be unethical and un-American. That is not the point, but we do believe that a tax of $5 is going to be prohibitive for the small dealer as well as the man that grows the crop, because he will average— I do not know what the average will be, but they raise as little as 2 acres.[22]

A representative for Chempaco and the Hemp Chemical Corporation raised similar objections.

The people making paper, and the finest grades of paper, which you cannot make in this country without the use of hemp at the present time . . . must have hemp fiber. . . . The paper manufacturer, when he gets the plant, simply blows [the] leaves away. They disappear when dried. They are gone. As a matter of fact, these people . . . did not know until two months ago that the hemp which they grew there contained marihuana. Until this agitation came up they did not dream of it.

Despite these pleas for common sense, the subcommittee seemed to have its mind made up. The bill was returned to the House with some suggestions, which were adopted and returned after being passed without a roll call. The Senate passed the bill without serious deliberation. President Franklin Roosevelt delivered the final blow with the stroke of a pen, when he signed the Marihuana Tax Act on 2 August 1937. Hemp, the environment, and the American farmer had lost. The corporate giants had won. But the crusade against hemp had only begun.

7

HEMP
FOR
VICTORY

I n the 1980s a fourteen-minute film began making the rounds in the hemp community. Titled *Hemp for Victory,* the film seemed to have been made by the United States Department of Agriculture (USDA) in 1942. It urged American farmers to grow hemp to support the war ef-

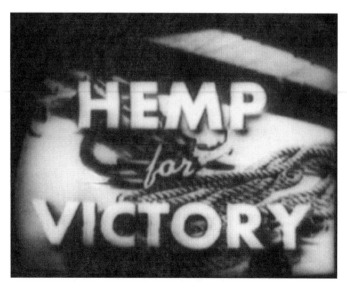

AN IMAGE FROM THE 1942 FILM *HEMP FOR VICTORY.*

fort with lines like "American hemp will go on duty again— hemp for mooring ships, hemp for tow lines, hemp for tackle and gear, hemp for countless naval uses both on ship and shore!" The Japanese had cut off America's supply of imported hemp, 34,000 feet of which was necessary for every battleship; nothing could be more patriotic, the film implied, than to grow acres of hemp for your country.

But could the USDA really have made a film heralding the merits of *Cannabis sativa,* when for years the government had waged a war to destroy the plant? If the film was legitimate, the official position that hemp was an "assassin of youth" with no place in society would be seriously compromised.

The United States government denied ever having made such a film. It must be a hoax, was the general consensus. Jack Herer and other activists asked every agency they could think of about the film and were met with the same answer, typified by this response from John Van Calcar of the Agricultural, Stabilization, and Conservation Service:

> We contacted the Washington DC office of the Department of Agriculture and also the Federal Audio Center and have been unable to locate any film with the title "Hemp for Victory" that was produced by any department of the federal government.

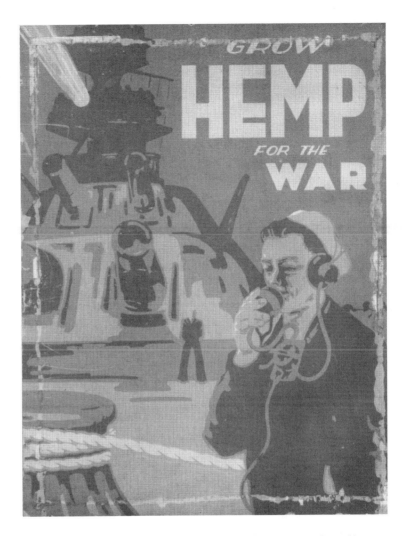

A WORLD WAR II U.S. GOVERNMENT POSTER. COURTESY OF OHIO HEMPERY.

Undeterred, Herer, Carl Packard, and Maria Farrow made their own search of the USDA library in Beltsville, Maryland. No record of *Hemp for Victory* was found. If any such film had ever been made, they were assured, it would be there. Next they made an exhaustive search of both the modern card catalogs and electronic files of the Library of Congress's motion pictures and filmstrips records, to no avail. Again, the librarians assured them that a listing could not simply disappear.

Concluding that a record of the film did not exist, Herer, Packard, and Farrow began to leave, when Herer had a final idea. Where would I have looked, he asked the

The general public was informed about the situation in *Newsweek* magazine's 16 October 1942 issue, in an article headlined simply "Hemp":

> Part of the cargo on the *Mayflower* was hemp seed. And, being the raw material for making rope and burlap, it was an important crop in this country all during the sailing ship era. But about the turn of the century it was replaced by imports of Manila hemp, sisal, and jute from Africa and the Orient.
>
> Long-range planners now are looking to the future even though present stockpiles will last until about 1944. Already the government has contracted for almost all the Haitian output of sisal, and that little republic is increasing its production. Last week the War Production Board approved plans for planting in the United States 300,000 acres of hemp (the only one of the fibers which will grow in this climate) and for building 71 processing mills. Plantings will be concentrated in Kentucky, Indiana, Illinois, Wisconsin, Minnesota, and Iowa, with the processing plants in approximately the same areas.
>
> This program should assure an adequate supply by the time stocks run out, for hemp is normally only a four-month crop. Farmers like it, too, because it helps control weeds, needs no tending until harvest, and leaves the soil in good condition.

librarian, if I had come here in the 1940s or 1950s? You wouldn't have sent me to the electronic files.

Of course not, the librarian said, you would have looked in the old card catalogs. Do you throw those out? asked Herer. No, we still have them, said the librarian, and she took Herer to the room that housed them. And there, in the dusty files, Herer found the following listing:

Hemp for Victory (Motion Picture)
U.S. Dept. of Agriculture, 1942.
14 min., sd., b&w, 16 mm.
  Summary: Explains that the war cut off the supply of East Indian coarse fibers, and stresses the need for American-grown hemp for military and civilian uses. Portrays farm practices of hemp growers in Kentucky and Wisconsin.
——Another issue. 35 mm.
  1. Hemp—U.S. 1. U.S. Dept. of
                    Agriculture.
                    633.53 Fi E 53–370
U.S. Office of Education. Visual Education Service

One can only wonder who made the decision to "delete" *Hemp for Victory* from the numerous official listings and what else has disappeared from the Library of Congress.

It seems that the "rewriting" of Official History, something we assume only occurs in communist Russia and other non-democratic states, is happening under our very noses.

Since Herer's discovery, patriotic citizens have helped turn up an abundance of resources detailing the U.S. Goverment's push to grow hemp during World War II. The United States Department of Agriculture has agreed that they made the film, and two copies have been registered with the Library of Congress.[1]

The irony of the United States being forced to grow hemp as a matter of national security must have galled Harry Anslinger, for just the previous year Anslinger had managed to have the term "cannabis" deleted from the official United States Pharmacopoeia and National Formulary. But not even the racists, industrial giants, and old-boy politicians who benefited from hemp's banishment could stand in the way of national defense, and hemp was badly needed, not just for rope and twine but for firehose, parachute webbing, and the shoelaces worn by every American soldier. When a young George Bush, who would later become president of the United States and Commander-in-Chief of the War on Drugs, parachuted from his plane into the Pacific in World War II, he dangled from a hempen lifeline.

So it was that in 1942 the federal government sponsored a crash program to produce enough hemp fiber to meet America's needs. A booklet titled *Hemp: A War Crop* brought farmers up to date with methods by which thousands of acres in the Midwest would be planted and new factories built to handle the crop: "Hemp growing in the U.S., which the Bureau of Narcotics in the past has tried to stop in order to prevent marijuana addiction, is now apparently going to be allowed and even encouraged as a result of the war."[2] Hemp seed was supplied to twenty thousand contracted farmers, with further instructions from the federally financed War Hemp Industries. Forty-two processing mills were built and equipped at a cost of $360,000 each by the Defense Plant Corporation.

Even children were enlisted in the wartime efforts to increase domestic hemp production. The University of Kentucky's agricultural extension service published a pamphlet, "The Hemp Seed Project for 4-H Clubs," which informed young patriots that "Uncle Sam has asked Kentucky to produce . . . the hemp seed for the nation." Encouraging 4-H members to serve their country during wartime, the booklet promised that labor requirements would not interfere with school work. Unfortunately for those who decided to fall in step with the government's

···

From *Hemp for Victory:*

Long ago when these ancient Grecian temples were new, hemp was already old in the service of mankind. For thousands of years, even then, this plant had been grown for cordage and cloth in China and elsewhere in the East. For centuries prior to about 1850 all the ships that sailed the western seas were rigged with hempen rope and sails. For the sailor, no less than the hangman, hemp was indispensable.

A 44-gun frigate like our cherished Old Ironsides took over 60 tons of hemp for rigging, including an anchor cable 25 inches in circumference. The Conestoga wagons and prairie schooners of pioneer days were covered with hemp canvas. Indeed the very word "canvas" comes from the Arabic word for hemp. In those days hemp was an important crop in Kentucky and Missouri. Then came cheaper imported fibers for cordage—like jute, sisal and Manila hemp—and the culture of hemp in America declined.

But now with Philippine and East Indian sources of hemp in the hands of the Japanese, and shipment from India curtailed, American hemp must meet the needs of our army and navy as well as of our industry. In 1942, patriotic farmers at the government's request planted 36,000 acres of hemp seed, an increase of several thousand percent. The goal for 1943 is 50,000 acres of hemp seed. . . .

This is hemp seed. Be careful how you use it, for to grow hemp legally you must have a federal registration and tax stamp. Ask your county agent about it. Don't forget . . . Hemp for Victory!

···

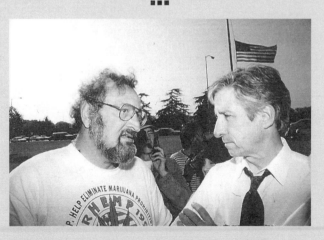

JACK HERER, LEFT, SPEAKING WITH SENATOR TOM HAYDEN. PHOTOGRAPH BY BILL BRIDGES.

new policies, the public mandates to grow hemp ended as suddenly as they had started. By 1944 the War Production Board felt confident that European suppliers could satisfy U.S. requirements, and responded by abruptly scaling down domestic production. As the war drew to a close, the government's stance on hemp once again flip-flopped. The patriotic crop, this wartime wonder-plant that held the promise of American victory, became the demon weed that would expose the republic to the communist threat.

The Reign of Law

As the era of McCarthyism dawned and all across America alternative lifestyles became suspect, the law's stranglehold on hemp tightened. A congressman from New York State introduced a bill in 1951 proposing the death penalty for violators of federal narcotics laws; a more lenient New York congressman suggested a minimum sentence of one hundred years. Senate hearings were held in 1951 in reaction to a perceived increase in drug use, especially among young men. Marijuana was accused of causing heroin addiction, and heroin was said to be

part of a communist plot to destroy America.

During the course of Senate hearings on a potential narcotics act, fifteen of the twenty-seven addicts who testified stated that marijuana was the first substance they had used before graduating to heroin. Several other "expert witnesses" affirmed a connection between marijuana and heroin.[3] The few dissenting voices included jurists who felt that mandatory minimum sentencing deprived the courts of the judicial discretion basic to American law. When the House debated the bill, one congressman contended that some youthful first-time offenders might suffer unduly, to which another congressman replied with a woefully misguided prophecy: "The enforcing officers will always have sympathy for the unfortunate consumer, especially if he is harmless. These enforcing officers are going to protect the high school boys and girls before the criminal courts until they know that they are collaborating with the peddlers."[4] Despite some debate on the issue, Congress passed the Boggs Act on 2 November 1951, increasing the penalties for all "narcotics" violations, including marijuana, to provide uniform penalties for the Marihuana Tax Act and the

Narcotic Drugs Import and Export Act.

Not all bureaucrats supported the passage of the act. James Bennett, director of the U.S. Bureau of Prisons, addressed judges at a conference of the fifth circuit in 1954, arguing that "the Boggs Bill was passed due to hysteria" and suggesting it violated the constitutional principle of the separation of powers. Displeased by this disagreement, Commissioner Anslinger assigned FBN agents to follow Bennett and report on his public statements and those of his associates. The fifth judicial circuit, however, took Bennett's advice and appointed a committee that unanimously recommended that the law be amended by removal of the provisions for mandatory minimum sentences. An irate Congressman Boggs criticized the dissenting judges: "I cannot imagine a more shortsighted recommendation. Anyone who has studied the narcotics trade and has seen the pitiful effect in countless homes throughout this nation from youths to the very old must recognize that this is one of the most vicious things in our country." Apparently others agreed with Boggs's assessment, for the Narcotic Control Act of 1956 passed through Congress with little de-

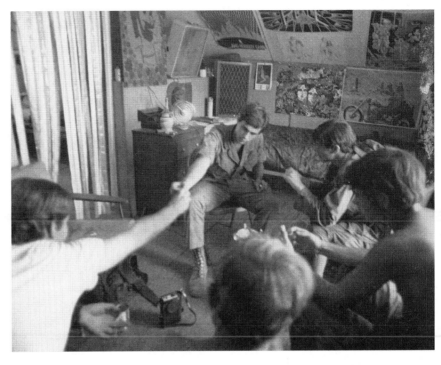

U.S. GIs PASS AROUND A JOINT. QUANG TRI PROVINCE, SOUTH VIETNAM, 1971.

bate or public attention, increasing the harshness of federal penalties for possession and sale of illicit substances.

Don't Trust Anyone Over Thirty

The decade of the 1960s opened with hemp occupying an ambiguous political and social position. Use of the mind-altering plant was becoming increasingly common, and some politicians were beginning to question the draconian policies of the previous decade. And yet legislation was not seriously considered as an option.

The United Nations adopted a policy on narcotics in 1961 stating that each member nation could adopt "such measures as may be necessary to prevent misuse of, and illicit traffic in, the leaves of the cannabis plant," and that "the use of cannabis (hemp) for other than medical and scientific purposes must be discontinued as soon as possible, but in any case within 25 years."[5] The U.S. Congress, which did not ratify the convention until 1967, seemed unsure of how to proceed.

By 1962 President John F. Kennedy had established an ad hoc group to study narcotic and substance abuse that ultimately announced:

> It is the opinion of the Panel that the hazards of marihuana per se have been exaggerated and that long criminal sentences imposed on an occasional user or possessor of the drug are in poor social perspective. Although Marihuana has long held the reputation of inciting individuals to commit sexual offenses and other antisocial acts, the evidence is inadequate to substantiate this.[6]

The next year, the President's Advisory Commission on Narcotics and Drug Abuse drew a clear distinction between cannabis and opiates, stating that unlawful sale or possession of marijuana was a less serious offense than the unlawful sale or possession of an opiate. Following President Kennedy before him, President Lyndon B. Johnson's Commission on Law Enforcement and Administration of Justice also rejected the "gateway" theory of marijuana-to-heroin use although hemp use was certainly not considered harmless. Unfortunately, a few more reasonable studies of cannabis use did not turn the tides of opinion. The majority of politicians and lawmakers maintained that hemp was a dangerous narcotic.[7]

While the marijuana-heroin connection continued to be gospel to many narcocrats and politicians, the hippies of the 1960s were learning for themselves that cannabis was not addictive and did not necessarily lead to heroin addiction. The very act of taking cannabis for the first time itself transformed consciousness, exclusive of any pharmacological properties of the plant. Young people discovered that they could smoke cannabis and nothing terrible would happen to their minds or bodies. In fact, the high didn't remotely incapacitate them the way liquor pirated from their parents' cabinets did. So what did that say about the other cautions and beliefs their parents and other purveyors of Establishment dogma had tried to pound into them? "Don't trust anyone over thirty" went the popular slogan, but the subtext was "Don't trust anyone who doesn't turn on." Since 1937, despite popular fear of marijuana, use of marijuana had nonetheless been spreading across the entire spectrum of society and was no longer confined to so-called marginal populations.

By the end of the sixties, marijuana had become a powerful political symbol of liberty and civil disobedience. "Smoking pot makes you a criminal and a revolutionary," said activist Jerry Rubin, speaking in May 1970. "As soon as you take your first puff, you are an enemy of society." In fact, the juggernaut of drug laws was used as a general weapon to crush political dissenters. FBI director J. Edgar Hoover directed a memo to all field offices in 1968: "Since the use of marijuana and other narcotics is widespread among members of the New Left, you should be alert to opportunities to have them arrested by local authorities on drug charges." One notable case involved Lee Otis Johnson, a black militant activist

and head of the Houston branch of the Student Nonviolent Coordinating Committee (SNCC). Johnson was sentenced by a Texas court to thirty years in prison for having given one joint to an undercover agent, a politically motivated conviction that was overturned by a federal district court in 1972.[8]

Tough laws might have been in force at home, but American troops in Vietnam were smoking potent marijuana to alleviate a dismal situation. The use of cannabis was more than common during the war; it was nearly universal. One well-known writer on the war beat reported that 75 percent of the soldiers stationed in Vietnam had used cannabis.[9] Some soldiers smoked cannabis habitually because it helped them overcome fear—that is, they felt it made them better soldiers. But others smoked it for precisely the opposite reason, as writer William Novak found when he interviewed veterans for his book *High Culture*. "We knew that stoned soldiers were not aggressive, alert, and effective soldiers," one veteran told him, "and because we opposed the war in a way that nobody but a grunt could experience, we used to say that smoking dope was a political statement . . . We enjoyed the idea that by getting high we

In contrast to public perception, even heroes smoked marijuana. The Associated Press reported on 22 June 1971: "A Congressional Medal of Honor winner says he was 'stoned' on marijuana the night he fought off two waves of Vietcong soldiers and won America's highest military honor."

He fought the enemy single-handed and dragged a wounded comrade to the rear before collapsing from exhaustion and three wounds. At a medical center, he refused treatment until more seriously injured men had been cared for.

"It was the only time I ever went into combat stoned," [the soldier] said. "You get really alert when you're stoned because you have to be. We were all partying the night before. We weren't expecting any action because we were in a support group. All the guys were 'heads.' We'd sit around smoking grass and getting stoned and talking about when we'd get to go home."

were frustrating the President, Westmoreland, and all those war-mongers in the rear."[10] When U.S. officials decided to abandon the war effort, the growing resistance of the fighting corps was a prime consideration. Soldiers were going AWOL, deserting, demonstrating, agitating, filing for conscientious-objector status, being insubordinate, mutinying, even rolling grenades into their officers' tents. Were marijuana and other drugs responsible for such determined opposition? Hardly—the war itself was a more vivid consciousness-raiser than any plant could be. But hemp undoubtedly helped raise the pitch of soldiers' awareness and bonded them to protesters back home.

In spite of the fact that cannabis use was widespread, political acceptance of the substance lagged far behind the social reality. The National Commission on Marihuana estimated that in 1971 up to 25 million Americans had used marijuana, but the official status of hemp held as many contradictions as ever. Several congressional committees had conducted hearings on the issue of drug control during 1969 and 1970, culminating in October of 1970 with the passage of the Comprehensive Drug Abuse Prevention and Control Act and the Controlled Substances Act, which established yet another commission. Chaired by Raymond Shafer, the National Commission on Marijuana and Drug Abuse recommended changes in the federal law. The commission suggested that the "possession of marihuana for personal use would no longer be an offense, but marihuana possessed in public would remain contraband subject to summary seizure and forfeiture. . . . Casual distribution of small amounts of marihuana for no remuneration or insignificant remuneration not involving profit would no longer be an offense."

Reacting against any such leniency, President Richard Nixon swore that he would fight against legalizing cannabis no matter what the commission recommended. In a message to Congress on 17 June 1971 he declared a "war on drugs." He depicted drug abuse as "a national emergency" and claimed that "if we cannot destroy the drug menace in the United States, then it will surely destroy us. . . . Drug traffic is public enemy number one domestically in the United States today and we must wage a total offensive, world-wide, nation-wide, government-wide, and if I may say so, media-wide."

As part of his war on drugs

President Nixon had established the Special Action Office for Drug Abuse Prevention and, more ominously, the Office for Drug Abuse Law Enforcement (ODALE). In shades of Watergate secret wiretaps were used, and "heroin hotlines" were set up to obtain anonymous tips by telephone. Federal officers began making street arrests of dealers and buyers, a trespass of authority that angered local law-enforcement agencies. Federal drug raiders sorely abused the "no-knock" provision (Title II) of the Comprehensive Drug Abuse Prevention and Control Act—which permitted officers to enter premises without a warrant or other notice if they believed that the drugs being sought would be destroyed or if someone's safety or life would be endangered by giving notice—and as a result this provision was repealed in 1974. The Bureau of Narcotics and Dangerous Drugs had been created by merging the Treasury Department's FBN with the Department of Health, Education, and Welfare's Bureau of Drug Abuse Control. Subsequently, Nixon's ODALE would merge with the Bureau of Narcotics and Dangerous Drugs and the Office of National Narcotics Intelligence in 1973 to form the Drug Enforcement Administration, the infamous DEA.[11]

President Ford was less strident than the Nixon administration concerning most of these issues. The Ford administration's Domestic Council Task Force released a White Paper on Drug Abuse in September 1975, which concluded that marijuana presents no serious potential harm to individuals and to society and recommended that federal efforts be focused instead on major trafficking cartels and manufacturers of heroin, barbiturates, and particularly amphetamines. However, the administration also supported some harsh efforts to eliminate the use of hemp, such as the poisoning of cannabis fields in Mexico.

The election of James E. Carter to the presidency in 1977 appeared to be a positive sign for those in favor of legalizing hemp. When he addressed Congress on 2 August 1977, President Carter became the first president to publicly endorse the decriminalization of marijuana. In his opinion, "Penalties against possession of a drug should not be more damaging to an individual than the use of the drug itself." Carter would have eliminated federal criminal penalties for the possession of up to one ounce of marijuana. The American Bar Association, the American Medical Association, the

In *Agency of Fear* Edward J. Epstein documents how the Nixon administration established ODALE and ultimately the DEA as a "private police force" to side-step the CIA and the FBI. According to Epstein the DEA was the final stage of the

White House timetable for consolidating its power over the investigative agencies of the government.... If the Watergate burglars had not been arrested and connected to the White House strategists, the DEA might have served as the strong investigative arm for domestic surveillance that President Nixon had sought. It had the authority to request wiretaps and no-knock warrants, and to submit targets to the Internal Revenue Service; and, with its counterintelligence agents, it had the talent to enter residences surreptitiously.

Two years after the DEA was established, a Senate subcommittee charged high-ranking officials in the agency with corruption, cover-ups, and mismanagement of money and personnel. Epstein writes that in Latin America, the DEA is widely considered to be a cover for covert CIA operations. DEA agents have created local drug vigilante groups by selecting, training, equipping, and paying the leaders and members. The teams sometimes arrest, torture, and illegally deport their fellow citizens to the United States for prosecution.[12]

■■■

The New York State Division of Substance Abuse Service developed a simple, accurate test for paraquat, although the test is not sensitive to very small amounts of the herbicide.

Soak and gently stir one gram of cannabis in one teaspoon of water for fifteen minutes. Strain the leaves to yield a brownish-yellow solution. Add one hundred milligrams of sodium bicarbonate and one hundred milligrams of sodium dithionate (available at photography stores). A blue-green color reaction indicates the presence of paraquat.

■■■

American Council of Churches, and other mainstream organizations joined in endorsing decriminalization. Such political sanity was obscured by scandal when Peter Bourne, director of the White House Office of Drug Abuse Policy, was forced to resign in 1978 after he wrote an illegal prescription for Quaaludes for one of his aides. Upon leaving the White House, Bourne told the press that there was "high incidence of marijuana use . . . [and] occasional use of cocaine" by staff members. The unsavory incident would later add fuel to the backlash against more lenient policies regarding hemp use, giving conservatives another excuse to oppose the so-called liberal approach.

ERADICATION

One of the most notorious elements of the DEA's war on drugs began during the Ford administration in 1976, when the U.S. government spent $60 million to fund a program of aerial spraying of hemp fields with paraquat, a nonselective contact herbicide that shrivels plants, giving them a sickly yellow tint and leaving a thin film of the mutagenic toxin. Even minute doses cause serious respiratory ailments such as fibrosis, lung lesions, intestinal disor-

ders, and convulsions. Higher doses cause irreversible kidney damage, respiratory failure, and death. Fully aware of these health risks, the DEA sent hundreds of aircraft and consultants to aid the ill-advised program that was sponsored by the Mexican federal government. The Carter administration terminated all funding for paraquat in September 1979, but Mexico continued to buy and use its own supplies, ignoring the potential dangers of using the poison.

Hemp farmers in Mexico apparently observed that the action of paraquat depends on sunlight and attempted to preserve their investment by harvesting immediately after the hemp was sprayed and wrapping it in dark cloths before exporting it to the United States. These homespun efforts were unsuccessful, and health risks awaited unsuspecting consumers. It was estimated that more than six thousand marijuana smokers were at risk of exposure to as much as five hundred milligrams of paraquat annually.[13]

The policy of spraying hemp crops with paraquat, halted temporarily by President Carter, was resumed during the Reagan administration. At the behest of President Ronald Reagan and with the support of Congress, the DEA again sprayed paraquat on hemp in national forests in Georgia, Kentucky, and Tennessee in 1983, despite public protests and a restraining order by U.S. District Court Judge Charles Moye. The Environmental Policy Act prohibits the use of paraquat in national forests. U.S. Representative Elliott Levitas called the spraying program "a dingbat idea" and estimated that the spraying, which cost nearly $1 million and involved only about sixty plants, cost $16,666 per plant. Money was no object, however; officials acknowledged that one reason for the spraying was to impress the Colombian government with American efforts to control cannabis by using paraquat and to convince them to do likewise. Georgia's Governor Joe Harris was not concerned about the potential health hazard to those who might smoke the poisoned plants, phrasing it thus: "We don't have any responsibility to those people. They are doing something illegal." Dr. Corey Slovis, director of emergency services at Grady Memorial Hospital in Atlanta, declared "the death penalty for smoking marijuana is too severe a penalty for anybody," but White House drug adviser Carlton E. Turner revealed the position of the Reagan administration, appearing on national television with the message that

■■■

During the paraquat panic of 1978, Carlton E. Turner was working for the University of Mississippi Marijuana Research Program, which was chartered to synthesize the psychoactive component in cannabis. At that time, Turner persistently tried to advertise a "paraquat tester" in High Times magazine. The magazine was not accepting ads for paraquat test kits because none had been proven to work. High Times associate editor Dean Latimer nonetheless entertained Turner's daily phone calls for a month, listening to Turner's sales pitch; he finally asked for a sample. Turner delivered a kit reminiscent of Rube Goldberg designs. Latimer wrote an article about the incident in 1984, showing Turner's fraudulent tester to be "just like the dozen or so phony kits other companies tried to buy ad space for at this time."

Turner went on to become the White House "drug czar" under President Reagan in 1981. By April 1985 Turner's conservative views magnified when he called for the

death penalty for drug dealers in his address at a PRIDE conference in Atlanta, Georgia, which Nancy Reagan and Imelda Marcos attended. He resigned in December 1986 after being discredited in Newsweek and other publications for his assertions that drugs alter people's lifestyles, that smoking marijuana may lead to homosexuality, and that gay men who use marijuana are risking damage to their immune system and vulnerability to AIDS. (Turner had visited some drug-treatment centers and learned that about 40 percent of the patients had engaged in homosexual activity.) Newsweek added a note: "Dr. Stanley Weiss of the National Cancer Institute says that a preliminary study found no causative link between pot and AIDS." After his resignation, Turner went into business developing urine-testing programs with Robert DuPont and Peter Bensinger—both former directors of the National Institute on Drug Abuse.[15]

■■■

if anyone died from paraquat-poisoned hemp, it would be a just punishment.[14]

The Colombian government did, in fact, respond to U.S. pressure and began in July 1984 to spray hemp fields with glyphosate, another herbicide. About 23,500 acres of hemp were under cultivation, resulting in roughly 10,000 tons for export to the United States at a time when Colombia provided about 60 percent of the marijuana that entered the U.S. market. President Reagan wrote a letter of praise to Colombia's President Betancur, congratulating his government's "decision to undertake a national aerial herbicide spraying campaign against marijuana," and touting his efforts as "an example for all nations to follow."[16]

INTERDICTION

The "war on drugs" has indeed been a battle. The Posse Comitatus Act of 1878—passed to provide citizens with protection against government militarism—prohibits the use of federal troops to enforce civilian laws. But beginning in 1969 the Act was so consistently violated in the name of drug enforcement that it was amended in 1982 to allow the U.S. military to execute drug laws.

On 5 September 1989, in his first major televised speech after becoming president, George Bush promised to continue the war against drugs. Indeed, some three months later the United States invaded Panama in Operation Just Cause, for the purpose of ousting General Manuel Noriega and his

Panama Defense Forces—allegedly because drug trafficking threatened U.S. security. Noriega was brought to the United States for trial at a cost of more than one thousand lives and nearly $200 million.

The U.S. military participated in the secretive Operation Ghost Dancer the next year. Despite local protests, the Ninth Infantry Division was used to raid hemp crops in Oregon. Senator Mark Hatfield thought that launching "drug warfare" against the people of his state was a fine idea, offering assurance that "in no way is this to violate the civil rights of any individuals."[17]

William J. Bennett, President Bush's director of the Office of National Drug Control Policy, blamed Oregon's liberal laws, lack of prisons and police, for its failure in the war against drugs. Bennett crystallized the essence of his get-tough approach during an interview on the "Larry King Show" in 1989, announcing that he had "no moral problems with beheading drug dealers—only legal ones." The evils of the drug were perfectly clear as far as Bennett was concerned: "Marijuana smoking makes people stupid." Bennett urged the California legislature to recriminalize possession promptly.

Californians had already been

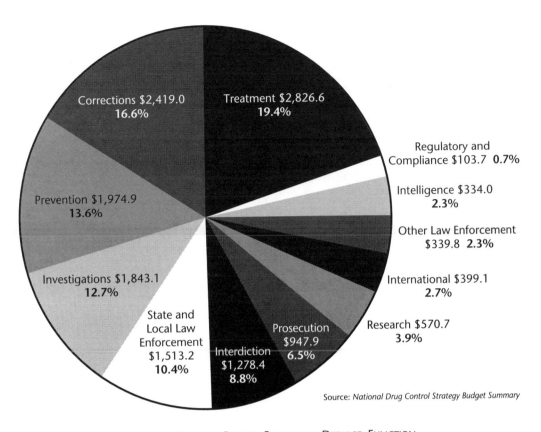

Source: *National Drug Control Strategy Budget Summary*

THE PRESIDENT'S FEDERAL DRUG CONTROL BUDGET REQUEST BY DETAILED FUNCTION, 1996 (DOLLARS IN MILLIONS). THE TOTAL BUDGET REQUEST: $14.6 BILLION. COMPARE THIS FIGURE TO THE DECISION BY THE U. S. HOUSE OF REPRESENTATIVES ON 19 SEPTEMBER 1995 TO OPEN THE PRISTINE ARCTIC NATIONAL WILDLIFE REFUGE TO OIL DRILLING BECAUSE IT WOULD GENERATE APPROXIMATELY $1/4$ BILLION DOLLARS IN REVENUE PER YEAR. IS THIS HOW YOU WANT YOUR TAX DOLLARS BEING SPENT?

treated to the Campaign Against Marijuana Planting (CAMP), funded by the state Bureau of Narcotics Enforcement and the federal DEA. CAMP troops destroyed hundreds of thousands of hemp plants, and President Reagan's Drug Policy Board gave CAMP a gold star for being such an excellent example of its national "cannabis suppression" strategy.[18] Several hundred formal complaints of civil-liberties abuses were filed against CAMP in federal court, charging that agents buzzed homes with helicopters and planes, held innocent people at gunpoint, invaded gardens and yards without search warrants, and in one case shot a family's dog. U.S. District Court Judge Robert Aquilar ruled in February

■■■

Parallel to government's attempt to eradicate hemp has been a campaign of propaganda to fix opinions in the minds of the nation's youth before they can form their own. The Le Dain Commission summarized the success of these efforts:

Many of the young people who have appeared before us have been critical of the drug education to which they have been exposed. In particular, they have said that the attempts to use 'scare tactics' have 'backfired' and destroyed the credibility of sound information. The conclusion we draw from the testimony we have heard is that it is a grave error to indulge in deliberate distortion or exaggeration concerning the alleged dangers of a particular drug, or to base a program of drug education upon a strategy of fear. It is no use playing 'chicken' with young people; in nine cases out of ten they will accept the challenge.

At times the techniques used by these propaganda groups seem to have more in common with a totalitarian regime than with the United States of America. In a 1991 DARE (Drug Abuse Resistance Education) program, an eleven-year-old girl told her instructor that her parents smoked marijuana. Police raided the home and arrested the couple. Also in 1991, a ten-year-old in Colorado did as instructed by a DARE officer and dialed 911 to report that there was marijuana in his house. The child then asked, "Can I come live at the police station?"[19]

■■■

1985 that CAMP agents "on numerous occasions [had] conducted warrantless searches and seizures" and committed "sustained and repeated buzzings, hoverings and dive bombing that at best disturb, and at worst terrorize, the hapless residents below," and ordered the agency to desist. Local activists organized to follow CAMP agents and catch them in violation of Judge Aquilar's order.

In October 1986 Agriculture Secretary Richard Lyng announced plans to create a five hundred person force, trained by the DEA or the FBI, to battle "heavily armed" hemp growers who had seized control of almost one million acres of national forests deemed "unmanageable" by the Forest Service. Congress authorized about $20 million for the effort and made hemp growing in national forests a federal felony.

Still battling the flow of marijuana between Mexico and the states nearly two decades after Operation Intercept, the U.S. provided twenty-four-hour coverage of the Arizona-Mexico border by National Guard units from four states for thirty days as part of Operation Harvest in 1987, during which time they identified ninety-three aircraft that fit the smuggling profile. National Guard or

Customs aircraft attempted to intercept a third of the targets, but only caught six, none of which carried any illegal substances. The operation cost $960,000. During an eighteen-day operation in May 1988, the U.S. Navy and U.S. Coast Guard used four destroyers and frigates to stop and board 35 ships out of 571 spotted by radar. They made only one marijuana seizure, worth about $400,000. The operation cost $6.5 million.

At the same time, the frustrated U.S. House of Representatives voted 385–23 to have the military seal the nation's borders and "substantially halt" the flow of illegal substances into the United States—within 45 days. The Defense Department submitted a job estimate of $22 billion and said that it would require 110 AWACS, 96 infantry battalions, 53 helicopter companies, 165 cruisers and destroyers, and 17 fighter squadrons. Defense Secretary Frank Carlucci told Congress the sobering truth about the plan in June 1988, calling it "a mission the armed forces cannot accomplish under any forseeable rules of engagement. . . . All the eradication and interdiction efforts in the world will not be effective as long as the demand for drugs in this country is so great."[20]

The achievements of decades of

"war" on hemp are difficult to measure—even for the government. In a 1983 report Government Accounting Office (GAO) auditors decried the unreliability of statistics on seizures used by law-enforcement agencies to gauge their drug-interdiction efforts. The GAO estimated that in 1981 the Customs Service overstated by 52 percent the amount of drugs it actually seized. Not until 1987 did the several agencies begin to assign identification numbers to the loads of drugs seized, to ensure that each load would be counted only once.[21] The GAO summarized seventeen years of the "drug war" in a 1988 report to Congress that stated flatly, "Our current approach is not working," and recommended working to reduce demand by emphasizing prevention, treatment, and research on the causes and extent of substance abuse. The office also observed that the so-called drug war had no leader. Instead, a patchwork of thirty-seven federal agencies attacked the problem without concert and fought each other in bureaucratic turf wars. President Reagan had vetoed a congressional plan to establish a single leader, but compromised by establishing a cabinet-level Drug Control Policy Board chaired by the U.S. attor-

ney general, the CIA director, and heads of the departments of Defense, State, Treasury, and Health. The GAO believed that the board had been ineffective, saying that it had been "unable to make the hard choices affecting agency budgets and programs necessary to bring cohesion to federal drug control efforts." The Anti-Drug Abuse Act of 1988 created a director of National Drug Control Policy, which allowed the likes of Carlton Turner and William Bennett to step forth as disparate heads of some sort of federal Hydra.[22] But the expense and confusion didn't end with this decision.

The National Drug Intelligence Center (NDIC) in Johnstown, Pennsylvania, opened for business in June 1993 for the purpose of consolidating the drug intelligence generated by nineteen different agencies. According to a critical report issued by the GAO, the $50 million facility is redundant and was a pork-barrel project for Senator John Murthas's hometown. The operations managers are located in Washington, D.C., because Johnstown is too far away from the decision-making center to be practical. The NDIC also duplicates work done at the El Paso Intelligence Center, established in 1974 with DEA funds and operated by representatives of thirteen

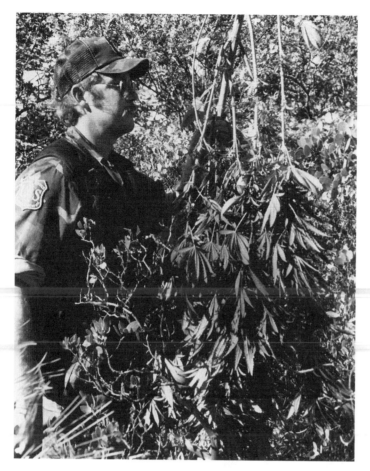

U.S. Forest Service ranger seizes "wild" hemp in Northern California. Photograph courtesy of USDA.

on the crime committed. Congress passed a series of crime and drug bills in the 1980s, imposing severe mandatory minimum sentences that soon caused a tripling of the nation's prison population. Drastic reverberations affected police work, lawyering, prosecution, prison standards, the judiciary, legislative intent, correctional theory, and public attitudes about hemp. A commission established in 1963 under Attorney General Robert F. Kennedy and President John F. Kennedy had urged for repeal of the severe mandatory sentences imposed by the Boggs Act and other legislation in the 1950s. The Kennedy report cited several negative effects that remain painfully apparent today: "prison crowding, outrageous prosecution, lack of judicial latitude, and an unchecked rise in violent crimes." In 1970 Congress had repealed all the mandatory sentences and restored the function of judicial discretion, but the problems didn't end there.

The Anti-Crime Bill of 1982 allowed judges to fine offenders for up to twice their profits and allowed the government to forfeit property in all felony drug cases. A fund was established with forfeiture proceeds to be used for further enforcement of drug laws. Each election year thereafter, the

federal agencies with agreements with all fifty states.[23]

MANDATORY MINIMUM SENTENCES

While various attempts have been made to eradicate hemp literally at the roots, additional efforts were made to give support to marijuana opposition by focusing

law became more repressive, resulting in the Crime Control Act
of 1984 and the Anti-Drug Act of
1986. A later mandate, The Anti-
Drug Act of 1988, declared as its
goal a "drug-free America," and
set 1995 as the target date for its
accomplishment. The act allowed
the death penalty for murders
committed in the course of a
drug-related felony, and required
individuals or contractors who buy
property or services worth twenty-
five thousand dollars or more
from any federal agency to certify
that they will provide a "drug-
free" workplace. Other laws
attempted to pressure states into
accepting federal definitions of
what constitutes a "drug" offense.
The 1990 Transportation Appro-
priations Act requires states to pass
laws revoking the driver's licenses
of people convicted of drug offenses for six months or else lose
millions of dollars in federal highway funds. On 27 June 1991, the
U.S. Supreme Court called drug
trafficking a grave threat to society and ruled that states may impose a life sentence without
parole for defendants convicted
for possession of large amounts of
controlled substances.[24]

One week after college basket-
ball star Len Bias—newly signed
with the Boston Celtics—died
from a cocaine overdose in 1986,

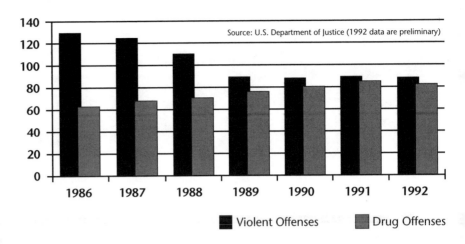

Source: U.S. Department of Justice (1992 data are preliminary)

Violent Offenses   Drug Offenses

AVERAGE FEDERAL SENTENCES FOR VIOLENT AND DRUG OFFENSES (IN MONTHS).

House Speaker Tip O'Neill, a
Democrat from Massachusetts, ordered the House crime subcommittee to draft a tough new drug
law that included longer mandatory minimum sentences. The results were questionable: Between
1950 and 1990 the average time
served for all serious non-drug
crimes fell by 65 percent while
drug sentencing rose sharply.
About 16 percent of the federal
prison population were drug offenders in 1970 and by 1994 the
proportion had risen to 62 percent, and was expected to reach
72 percent by 1997. While the
drug war has fueled a major crisis
in the prison system it has had
little effect on the drug problem:
the national prison population has
doubled since 1982, and even tripling prison capacity would not

Mandatory minimum sentences for cannabis offenders has overflowed our prisons, but not with the major dealers you might expect. Rather, a *Boston Globe* study of the eastern counties of Massachusetts found that first-time offenders accounted for 26 percent of the drug-offender prison population in 1994, up from just 2 percent in 1989. These small fry, in fact, often serve *more* time than the hard-core dealers. Why? Because of the rule by which agencies may seize drug-offenders' assets. Agencies have come to depend on these assets for a staggering 12 percent of their funding, even though, according to the *Globe,* only 43 percent of seized assets actually go toward fighting the war on drugs. Other assets have gone toward paying overtime, rent, and other unrelated expenses. But unless they are caught red-handed, dealers do not part with their assets so readily, so a system of authorized bribes takes place, with dealers "forfeiting" their assets in return for reduced sentences or parole.[25]

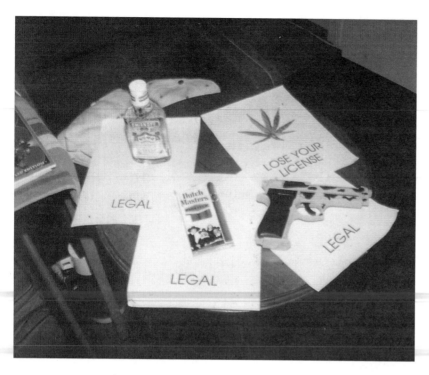

A QUESTIONABLE VALUE SYSTEM. PHOTOGRAPH BY BILL BRIDGES.

cause significant reduction in drug availability. In 1994 about two hundred thousand people were in state and federal prisons for drug offenses. Meanwhile, violent criminals have been freed from jail early to make room for nonviolent offenders, which leaves people like San Francisco Sheriff Michael Hennessey in despair: "Drug dealers and users have consumed the single most valuable resource in the criminal justice system: jail cells. We desperately need the limited space in our nation's jails and prisons to house violent offenders."

The injustice generated by mandatory minimum sentencing for drug offenses has moved nearly a hundred senior federal judges to refuse to hear such cases, and many other justices have retired prematurely for the same reason. In a recent survey of Massachusetts Superior Court Judges, 92 percent opposed mandatory minimums.[26] When New York Judge Jack Weinstein announced his decision to retire, he wrote, "I need a rest from the oppressive sense of futility that these drug cases leave. I simply cannot sentence another impoverished person whose destruction has no discernible effect on the drug trade."

| 18,000 | |
| 16,000 | |

Total Violent Crimes

Source: *The Boston Globe,* Sept. 27, 1995

Total Sentences for Violent Crimes (in months)

IN MASSACHUSETTS, VIOLENT CRIME GOES UP, BUT VIOLENT CRIMINALS ARE BACK ON THE STREET SOONER.

FORFEITURE

Law-enforcement officials have long been able to punish convicted criminals by confiscating their property, but it was not until 1984 that Congress authorized confiscation without first charging the individual with a crime. The drug-law provisions that allow seizure and forfeiture of cash and assets have been a goldmine for lawmen, but a nightmare for thousands of victims of civil rights abuses. Asset forfeiture and cash seizures make a mockery of civil rights and provide ample opportunity for corruption. The DEA has contended that 80 percent of people whose property they seize do not contest the action, thus "proving" that most of the assets appropriated are the fruit of criminal labor. Critics say

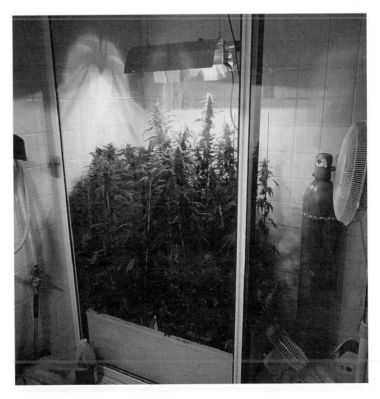

AS THE DEA GETS TOUGHER, HEMP GROWERS GET INNOVATIVE. PHOTOGRAPH BY ANDRE GROSSMAN.

The modern legislative form of "reefer madness" has caused tragedies far worse than any of the fantastic marijuana gore stories of the 1930s. In one extreme case—and there are many—the individual who suffered the consequences of overzealous law enforcement was Mark Young. Young merely introduced two marijuana dealers in Indianapolis who later did business together, were arrested, and cooperated with the government. They fingered Young, who received a life sentence without possibility of parole in February 1992.[27]

Also in 1992, Edward Czuprynski, a politically active attorney in Bay City, Michigan, was convicted in a federal court for possession of 1.6 grams of marijuana and was sentenced to fourteen months imprisonment. In a Michigan state court, he would have received a fine of one hundred dollars. Czuprynski's license to practice law was suspended, forcing his successful firm to go out of business. He spent almost eight months in prison before being released on appeal.[28]

James Cox, a cancer patient who grew hemp for use as an anti-emetic with his chemotherapy, was convicted for it in Missouri and sentenced to fifteen years in prison. Orland Foster, an AIDS patient who also grew hemp for medical purposes in North Carolina, served fifteen months for the same offense. Foster's cellmate served less time—for murder.

The case of paraplegic Jim Montgomery, who smoked marijuana to relieve his muscle spasms, is even more inhuman. Sheriffs in Sayre, Oklahoma, found two ounces of marijuana in the pouch on his wheelchair. He was convicted by a jury that sentenced him to life imprisonment plus sixteen years. The judge later reduced the sentence to ten years. He was released on appeal bond after nearly a year in a prison hospital, where he developed a life-threatening infection. The government also tried to forfeit Montgomery's home, which he shared with his widowed mother.[29]

collection for the agencies involved, and these agencies have become addicted to the money.

One of the most common abuses involves a legal "shakedown," whereby defendants buy their cars back from prosecutors. Civil forfeiture actions deprive suspects of their possessions while their criminal trials are pending, robbing them either of their defense funds or of vehicles needed to hold legitimate jobs. Some defendants decline to contest civil forfeitures because a person cannot take the Fifth Amendment in a civil case, and the civil testimony could damage the criminal case.[30]

An extreme violation of both civil rights and common sense occurred when the motor yacht *Ark Royal*, valued at $2.5 million, was seized when the Coast Guard found ten hemp seeds and two stems aboard the ship. Prompted by public criticism of the case, the ship was returned after the owner paid sixteen hundred dollars in fines. In a similar incident, the ninety-foot *Lorraine Carol* and its cargo (eleven tons of scallops) was seized by the Coast Guard in May 1988 when part of a marijuana cigarette and a few seeds were found in the crew's quarters. The felony charges against the ship's owner were later dropped, but the experience cost him twenty

that it only goes to show how difficult it is to recover property from the government. In fact, no criminal charges are filed in more than half of federal forfeiture cases. Rather, they argue that the primary purpose of the laws—to inflict suffering on alleged drug dealers—becomes secondary to revenue

thousand dollars in legal fees, eighty thousand dollars in lost income, and a two hundred and fifty dollar fine. In another unfortunate case, the DEA seized the home of Wayne and Ellen Treadway in 1989 after finding marijuana growing in a backyard shed. Wayne Treadway was convicted and served eleven months for a misdemeanor. The government sold the house and returned half of the proceeds to Ellen Treadway, who was left homeless with her three children and two foster children. Newspapers around the country have given many accounts of other horror stories resulting from these obscene laws, which yield about $1.5 billion worth of seized cash and property each year.[31]

■■■

At 9 A.M. on 2 October 1992 a thirty-person task force (including representatives from the Los Angeles Police Department, the DEA, the California National Guard, and the National Park Service) assaulted the two hundred-acre Trails End Ranch in Malibu, California. The ostensible reason for the raid was to seize hemp allegedly being cultivated on the property. The raiders shot and killed David Scott when he came armed with a pistol to the defense of his wife, who was screaming for help.

The search warrant was based on a federal agent's claim of having seen a hemp-growing operation while conducting aerial surveillance—without binoculars—from a thousand feet above the ground. The usual "reliable informant" also supported the claim; yet, no hemp plants, no marijuana, no paraphernalia, nor any related contraband whatsoever were found after the lawmen searched the property for several hours.

Donald Scott was heir to a large family fortune built on his grandfather's sales of Scott's Emulsion. The *Los Angeles Times* reported on 11 October 1992 that "Scott had refused on several occasions to sell his property to the state." After a five-month investigation, the Ventura County District Attorney concluded that the true motive for the raid was in fact to seize the ranch—valued at $5 million—under federal forfeiture laws. The government had obtained an appraisal of the property and included that information in the preraid briefing. The seizure of Scott's ranch was discussed at the same time, and agents stood by ready to take immediate possession of the property, had drugs been found.

■■■

INFORMANTS

The drug laws have also created a veritable industry of so-called confidential informants. In a particularly disturbing example, Sheriff Gene Taylor of Anderson County, South Carolina, encouraged residents to buy illicit substances to set up dealers, promising to pay them up to 25 percent of any money or assets seized in the arrest. The sheriff bought billboards advertising: NEED MONEY? TURN IN A DOPE DEALER. Anderson said, "I want people to realize they can make really good money, depending on how much they cooperate."[32]

Informing has become a mass occupation that manufactures crime and lies for personal gain. Hired informants often commit crimes to maintain their covers and can be granted immunity if caught. Police officers sometimes fabricate confidential informants so as to obtain search warrants, because judges almost never demand that the identity of the informant be revealed.[33] Entire cases are based on the unsubstantiated assertions of informants, sometimes with tragic results. On 26 August 1992 Donald Carlson, a forty-one-year-old computer-company executive, awoke near midnight at the sound of violent banging on his door. The intruders would not identify themselves, so Carlson called the police, then he fired two warning shots. The agents battered down the door, threw in a stun grenade, shot Carlson, then shot him twice again as he lay disarmed on the floor. No drugs were found. Authorities said that an informant "told wild tales" about heavily armed South American drug dealers using Carlson's suburban home as a cocaine warehouse. The informant was charged with lying to agents, and the authorities made a rare public apology.[34]

Likely no individual has malevolently plotted to bring about the destruction and misery caused by the War on Drugs. Instead, more and more individuals are caught up in an out-of-control effort to fix societal ills, and more and more lives are ruined in the name of morality. Aztec priests intended no evil as their cult slaughtered thousands in the name of the gods; they believed it necessary to preserve their culture. It didn't work. Like the Aztecs, our own priests of morality ruin an ever-increasing number of lives in their own version of human sacrifice, with the same purpose—to save a culture from itself—and with as little chance for salvation. The time has come to make a change.

Legalize It!

Which countries are legally growing hemp in 1995? Canada, Austria, France, Great Britain, The Netherlands, Poland, Hungary, Ukraine, Russia, Romania, India, China, Korea, and many others. Interest in hemp continues to explode. Hemp is here to stay, and it is already improving the environmental and economic health of dozens of nations. Ironically, the two nations with absolute obsessions for hemp products—the United States and Germany—still allow no domestic hemp production. Instead, local farms go bankrupt while these countries feed their dollars to countries able to grasp the difference between low-THC and high-THC hemp.

The easiest argument for the legalization of hemp in the United States (and any other country where it is still illegal) is to focus on industrial hemp alone. As this book has shown, you can't keep a good plant down. The sheer usefulness of the plant for industry, health, food, and the environment has overcome the campaigns of propaganda and eradication directed against it, and its true history is becoming better known every day. The only argument against industrial hemp in the United States has been that verdant waves of cannabis across a sizable chunk of the nation would make it excessively difficult for the DEA to do its job. This argument no longer holds weight. Studies by Paul Mahlberg and others indicate that it is possible to introduce morphological markers into high-fiber strains of hemp that would make it simple for law enforcement to distinguish between industrial hemp and psychoactive hemp. With this final roadblock removed, there is no reason to continue to deprive our farmers, soil, streams, economy, and citizens of industrial hemp. Case closed.[35]

But the legalization of industrial hemp is not enough. Is it the place to start? Definitely. The most important step? Unquestionably. But to allow ourselves to be appeased with hemp for jeans and paper while thousands of medical patients suffer needlessly and harmless citizens fill our jails would be to silently condone behavior that is crippling our society. Goverment's ban on hemp depends largely on

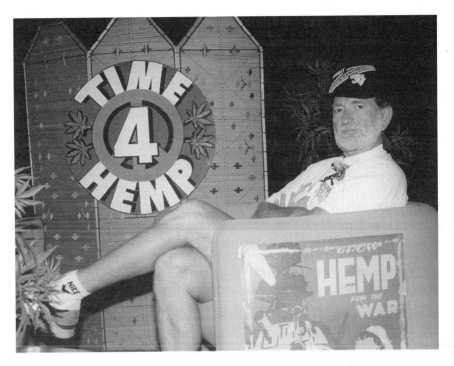

LONG-TIME HEMP ADVOCATE AND COUNTRY MUSIC SUPERSTAR WILLIE NELSON. PHOTOGRAPH BY BILL BRIDGES.

maintaining the ignorance of its citizens regarding the plant's history. If we are told hemp is a monster more hideous than Frankenstein, we will believe it unless we hear otherwise. But now we do know otherwise. The true history of hemp is out there for anyone to hear, and it would be a betrayal of our democratic ideals if we didn't push for absolute justice.

COMPASSIONATE CANNABIS

As the United States clings to what has been called a "patho-

> ■■■
> Hemp *is* legally grown in the United States. Exactly two permits to grow cannabis have been issued by the DEA. One of the recipients is Dr. Paul Mahlberg of Indiana University at Bloomington. Since 1970 Dr. Mahlberg has grown hemp to study cannabinoid-generation and morphology in the plant, with the aim of altering the THC gene in fiber hemp to unequivocally distinguish it from psychoactive hemp.
> ■■■

■■■

Stephen Jay Gould, the eminent Harvard paleontologist, gave testimony regarding the medical value of cannabis, reproduced in Dr. Lester Grinspoon and James Bakalar's 1993 book *Marijuana, the Forbidden Medicine*:

I am a member of a very small, very fortunate, and very select group— the first survivors of the previously incurable cancer, abdominal mesothelioma. . . . When I started intravenous chemotherapy (Adriamycin), absolutely nothing in the available arsenal of antiemetics worked at all. I was miserable and came to dread the frequent treatments with an almost perverse intensity.

I had heard that marihuana often works well against nausea. I was reluctant to try it because I have never smoked any substance habitually. . . . Moreover, I had tried marihuana twice (in the usual context of growing up in the sixties) and had hated it. (I am something of a Puritan on the subject of substances that, in any way, dull or alter mental states—for I value my rational mind with an academician's overweening arrogance. . . .) But anything to avoid nausea and the perverse wish it induces for an end of treatment.

The rest of the story is short and sweet. Marijuana worked like a charm. I disliked the "side effect" of mental blurring . . . but the sheer bliss of not experiencing nausea— and then not having to fear it for all the days intervening between treatments—was the greatest boost I received in all my year of treatment, and surely had a most important effect upon my eventual cure. It is beyond my comprehension—and I fancy I am able to comprehend a lot, including much nonsense—that any humane person would withhold such a beneficial substance from people in such great need simply because others use it for different purposes."[36]

■■■

logical political agenda" to suppress cannabis with lies and laws, perhaps its cruelest action is the continued refusal to reclassify marijuana for medical purposes. Countless numbers of people are deprived of access to an excellent medicine that can alleviate their suffering and can sometimes even treat their disease.

The Controlled Substances Act (CSA) of 1970 had placed marijuana under Schedule I, the most restrictive classification, thus making it unavailable for medical use. The National Organization for the Reform of Marijuana Laws (NORML) filed a petition with the Bureau of Narcotics and Dangerous Drugs in May 1972, urging the bureau to reclassify cannabis to Schedule II so doctors could prescribe it as a medicine. The petition was summarily rejected without holding public hearings as required by the CSA. It was falsely claimed that reclassification of cannabis would violate the obligations of the U.N. Single Convention on Narcotic Substances.

NORML was joined by the Alliance for Cannabis Therapeutics (ACT), which also filed thirteen "patient petitions" with the DEA. Again and again, NORML and ACT appealed for a review of their joint petition. After still more delaying inaction, the DEA saw fit to conduct hearings, fifteen years after the initial court order to that effect. The hearings were held from summer 1986 until summer 1988 (Docket No. 86-22).[37]

Administrative law judge Francis Young reviewed the documentary evidence and the testimonies of the many patients and doctors who appeared as witnesses, and on 6 September 1988 issued his sixty-nine-page ruling *In the Mat-*

ter of Marihuana Rescheduling Petition. He wrote, in part:

> Marijuana, in its natural form, is one of the safest therapeutically active substances known. . . . The cannabis plant considered as a whole has a currently accepted medical use in treatment in the United States. There is no lack of accepted safety for use under medical supervision and it may lawfully be transferred from Schedule I to Schedule II. The judge recommends the Administrator transfer cannabis. . . . The evidence in this record clearly shows that marijuana has been accepted as capable of relieving the distress of great numbers of very ill people, and doing so with safety under medical supervision. It would be unreasonable, arbitrary and capricious for the DEA to continue to stand between those sufferers and the benefits of this substance in light of the evidence in this record. . . . In strict medical terms, marijuana is far safer than many foods we commonly consume."

DEA administrator John Lawn rejected the court's decision. "Accounts of these individuals' suffering and illnesses are very moving and tragic. They are not, however, reliable scientific evidence. These stories of individuals who treat themselves with a mind-altering drug, such as marijuana, must be viewed with great skepticism." In 1989 Lawn charged that advocates of medical cannabis had a "Dark Ages" mentality and had "attempted to perpetrate a dangerous and cruel hoax on the American public."[38]

Witnesses who testified before the DEA hearings held from 1986 to 1988 repeatedly emphasized that cannabis does indeed have a crucial medicinal purpose, and that prohibition is not only unfounded but unfair. Dr. William Regelson said, "I have other things to do than waste my time with stupid fears of a physician-mediated 'plague' for what should be a controlled substance of some value. Do we have major problems with physician abuse of morphine, methadone, demerol, codeine, etc.? The problem is a psycho-social issue resembling the search for witches of an earlier era. Preventing a psychoactive drug's entry into Schedule II will not solve crime on our streets and hurts patients who can benefit from an expanded therapeutic option."[39]

In April 1991 the appeals court decided that Lawn "had acted with a vengeance" to reject Judge Young's recommendation, and it ordered the DEA to restudy its opposition to marijuana. The DEA demanded that cannabis must meet a new set of impossible standards for accepted medical use, based on the Food, Drug and Cosmetic Act. The plaintiffs appealed once more, and in April 1991 a three-judge panel of the U.S. Courts of Appeals ordered the DEA to reconsider its opposition to marijuana as medicine and to re-evaluate its criteria, which were considered illogical and impossible to satisfy. Again, the DEA refused to act, and in March 1992 it issued its final rejection of any petitions to reschedule cannabis. On 18 February 1994, the U.S. Court of Appeals upheld the DEA decision to keep marijuana classified as a Schedule I substance.[40]

Meanwhile, in May 1991 the United Nations reassigned THC from Schedule I (as established by the 1971 Convention on Psychotropic Substances) to Schedule II, because the pure substance has been proven useful for several medical purposes, and it is "not widely used outside legitimate medical channels." The cannabis plant, however, remained in Schedule I, because it is "used illegally by millions of people worldwide." In a classic case of bureaucratic reverse-logic, this means that the natural plant, growing wild or cultivated, is anathema, but if the powerful chemical THC, which is what makes hemp illegal in the first place, is extracted from the roots, leaves, fiber, cellulose, etc., then this concentrated drug—with an exorbitant price due to research and development—is suddenly granted legal venues.

A parallel effort to bypass the Controlled Substances Act began in 1975, when Robert C. Randall, a glaucoma patient, was arrested for cultivating cannabis. He sustained a defense of "medical necessity," since THC is proven to reduce intraocular pressure (IOP) in glaucoma with negligible side-effects when other conventional treatments have failed. More than 7000 Americans go blind from glaucoma each year; more than 250,000 people in the United States suffer from the incurable disease, and so do millions more worldwide. Being obliged to supply Randall with licit medicinal marijuana, the U.S. government created the Compassionate Investigative New Drug (IND) program, through which qualified patients could obtain their supply. The application process involved a ludicrous amount of paperwork, and few doctors were willing to take on the task.[40]

Beginning with New Mexico in 1978, thirty-five states passed legislation by overwhelming majorities to allow the medicinal use of cannabis. The NIDA processed and distributed more than 160,000 marijuana cigarettes for human use between 1976 and 1990. In June 1991 Herbert Kleber, the deputy director of National Drug Control Policy, assured the public that anyone with a legitimate medical need for cannabis would be able to receive a Compassionate IND. Yet, only about fifty persons ever were approved for the program, and James Mason, chief of the Public Health Service under the Bush administration, cancelled the program entirely in March 1992 after a surge of new applications from AIDS patients.

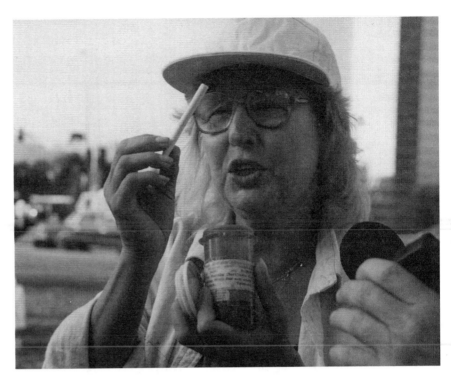

ELVY MUSIKKA, THE FIRST AMERICAN FOR WHOM CANNABIS WAS LEGALLY PRESCRIBED, HOLDING A U.S. GOVERNMENT JOINT. PHOTOGRAPH BY BILL BRIDGES.

In defense of its position, Drug Enforcement Agency Administrator Robert Bonner said, "Claims of marijuana's medical benefits are a cruel hoax to offer false hope to desperate people," and he compared the modern movement to support the medical use of cannabis to a time when, "a century ago, many Americans relied on snake oil salesmen to pick their medicines."

In July 1994 the Public Health Service announced that it would not lift the ban on cannabis. Assistant Health Secretary Philip Lee wrote: "Sound scientific studies supporting these claims are lacking despite anecdotal claims that smoked marijuana is beneficial," but the PHS may allow privately funded experiments to determine if cannabis has any health benefits.[41]

Although the use of cannabis as a medicine has been criticized because the notorious "euphoric" effects of THC allegedly detract from its therapeutic virtue, the word "euphoria" means "a sense of well-being," which is vital to the healing process. Other witnesses at the 1986–1988 DEA hearings defended marijuana in this regard.

This Policy Is Evil

Janet Andrews testified to the DEA that her young son Josh, a cancer patient, "successfully used marijuana for two years without ever encountering one serious adverse physical effect."

By comparison, the chemotherapy drugs he used destroyed his immune system, damaged his one remaining kidney, and caused all of his hair to fall out. Is marijuana"safe"? Compared to what? Certainly, marijuana is far "safer" than the drugs currently approved as safe by the FDA for anticancer treatments. . . .

Josh also suffered no serious mental problems as a result of his therapeutic use of marijuana. The much-discussed marijuana "high" certainly did not cause him any problems and, to a significant extent, was actually helpful. I particularly remember Josh giggling once shortly after receiving his chemotherapy. Giggling—is that an "adverse effect"? In the next room, a child without marijuana was fighting for his breath while vomiting up bile.

Josh is now 10 years old. He sur-

vived. His one percent chance has become a lifetime. Marijuana made the difference between life and death for Josh. But, even if things had not turned out so well, even if Josh had died as a result of his cancer and his chemotherapy, marijuana would still have made a significant contribution to his welfare. There is life and death. And there is suffering. Marijuana may not "save" a patient from death, but it makes the life which remains far more worth living. . . .

There were times during Josh's treatment when the sheer madness and meanness of the law overwhelmed me. Why would the government allow Josh's doctors to prescribe morphine, but not marijuana? It is perfectly legal to pump my four-year-old son full of extraordinarily toxic chemotherapy drugs, but God forbid anyone should try to legally provide him with a much safer drug, like marijuana! This policy is so stupid, so insensitive to human needs and legitimate medical treatment, it is evil.

In his testimony to the DEA, cancer patient John Dunsmore III said, "I've never had an adverse reaction to marijuana. Usually I have a good time. Euphoria isn't necessarily a bad thing. Marijuana allows me to get out of myself, to think about myself in a different,

more detached way. It helps me feel relaxed. Feeling relaxed when you're fighting for your life helps you fight."

Thomas Jefferson and Dr. Benjamin Rush, who was George Washington's personal physician and a signer of the Declaration of Independence, both foresaw that the federal government might attempt to control medicine. Dr. Rush warned that unless medical freedom was constitutionally guaranteed, medicine would eventually become "an undercover dictatorship," in which the art of healing would be restricted to one class of men while equal privileges were denied to others. "The Constitution of this republic should make special privilege for medical freedom as well as religious freedom," Rush argued, but to no avail, and, unfortunately, his prophecy has come true.

Even less reason exists to maintain the ban on medical cannabis than exists to ban industrial hemp. The evidence of cannabis's potential to relieve nausea and pain is substantial, and no one—not doctors, scientists, or politicians—claims that cannabis is more potent than morphine. Morphine is legally prescribed and abuse has not been a major problem. If this and other strong narcotics can be placed on Schedule

II, why not cannabis? Not until the sound of this question being asked is deafening can we hope that the government will face the truth of hemp's healing properties.

DECRIMINALIZATION

Many activists within the hemp community do not like to mix industrial hemp issues with psychoactive cannabis issues. Psychoactive substances are a much stickier issue, while industrial hemp is a simple matter of economics, environmental health, and common sense. But the injustices being perpetrated on our citizens—both the ones serving jail time and the rest of us forced to foot the bill for the War—are as vile as the injustices being done to our planet by industry. In the past thirty years, a growing number of voices has objected.[42]

The public movement to legalize cannabis can be said to have begun on 16 August 1964 when a young man walked into a San Francisco police station, lit a joint, and asked to be arrested. His attorney, James R. White III, subsequently formed LeMar (LEgalize MARijuana), which sponsored the first demonstrations against marijuana laws in America in Union Square that December.

For a time progress toward

▪▪▪
The Le Dain Commission

The Canadian government appointed a commission of inquiry into the non-medical use of drugs in May 1969. It was popularly called the Le Dain Commission after its chairman, Gerald Le Dain, dean of Osgoode Hall Law School at York University in Toronto. In its 320-page interim report, which appeared April 1970, the commission described the need to legalize the simple possession of cannabis (and other psychotropics) in terms of the cost of prohibition. Enforcement of drug laws, the commission said, cost far too much in individual and social terms including "the destruction of young lives and growing disrespect for law." The commission suggested that the present law against simple possession of cannabis was probably unenforceable.

The Commission is of the opinion that no one should be liable for imprisonment for simple possession of a psychotropic drug for non-medical purposes. . . . The illicit status of cannabis invites exploitation by criminal elements, and other abuses such as adulteration; it also brings cannabis users into contact with such criminal elements and with other drugs, such as heroin, which they might not otherwise be induced to consider. . . . For all of these reasons, it is said, cannabis should be made available under government-controlled conditions of quality and availability.[44]

▪▪▪

---

legalization seemed to gain momentum. Between 1967 and 1974 the federal government and all the states except Nevada reduced the simple possession of marijuana to a misdemeanor. The reason was simple: many thousands of children of respectable families were being arrested for possession of marijuana and stigmatized with a criminal record. Parents did not want their children to suffer throughout life because of a trivial youthful folly, and they acted accordingly.[43]

In 1975 Alaska's Supreme Court

NORML

The National Organization for the Reform of the Marijuana Laws was established by Keith Stroup in 1970. Since then, NORML has lobbied on the state and federal levels to persuade America's legislators to legalize cannabis. The group shifted its emphasis from lobbying to education in 1983. Director Don Fiedler responded in 1990 to the misconception that the organization is generally "pro drugs":

The fact is we are the National Organization for the Reform of Marijuana Laws, and it's not appropriate we get caught in the backlash of all the fervor resulting from the crack epidemic in this country. Our position, very simply, is we know it makes absolute and total sense to consider regulations for marijuana, with appropriate licensing, with advertising bans, with taxation and age, time, and place restrictions. And by doing that we will have helped, either directly or indirectly, with the drug problem in our country.[45]

decided in *Ravin v. State* that possession and personal use of cannabis by adults at home was a constitutionally protected private activity with so little impact on society that the state is not entitled to interfere. The court issued a fifty-four-page opinion that said, "It appears that effects of marijuana on the individual are not serious enough to justify widespread concern, at least as compared with the far more dangerous effects of alcohol, barbiturates, and amphetamines." The law stood until 1990, when it was rescinded by a narrow voting margin after the Bush administration threatened to withhold federal highway funds from Alaska if the state did not recrim-inalize cannabis.

By the late 1970s, it was apparent that those states which had decriminalized cannabis had not collapsed into chaos. The Drug Abuse Council commissioned four surveys in Oregon which determined that the use of marijuana had increased only slightly by 1978, and the majority of adults in the state favored further relaxation of the law. The costs of law enforcement and criminal justice were noticeably reduced. By 1980 only eleven states had eliminated criminal penalties for possession of cannabis, but they were big states—representing nearly one-third of the total population of the United States. The Addiction Research Foundation surveyed the literature of the period and concluded that "decriminalization of marijuana does not appear to have had a major impact on the rates of use, as many people feared it might. . . . It would appear that decriminalization measures have succeeded in reducing the costs of law enforcement without substantially increasing the health and safety hazards."[46]

In his address to Congress in 1977, President Carter had become the first president to publicly endorse decriminalization of marijuana; nearly five years later—after four years of study—the prestigious National Academy of Sciences (NAS) released *An Analysis of Marijuana Policy*. The forty-one-page report analyzed the "social costs" of enforcing the criminal laws against marijuana use and concluded that the laws against marijuana fail to deter millions of users and lead to the "consequent criminalization of large numbers of young Americans." The panel noted that in California, the decriminalization of marijuana had resulted in a 74 percent reduction in costs of enforcing the cannabis laws. The committee recommended more public discussion about legalizing and regulating the sale of marijuana, adding that

> there is reason to believe that widespread uncontrolled use would not occur under regulation. Indeed, regulation might facilitate patterns of controlled use by diminishing the "forbidden fruit" aspect of the drug and perhaps increasing the likelihood that an adolescent would be introduced to the drug through families and friends, who practice moderate use, rather than through their heaviest-using, most drug-involved peers.[47]

The National Drug Control Strategy issued by the White House in 1989 stated that "legalizing drugs would be an unqualified national disaster. In fact, any significant relaxation of drug enforcement—for whatever reason, however well-intentioned—would promise more use, more crime, and more trouble for desparately [sic] needed treatment and education efforts," according to "drug czar" William Bennett.

Speaking at Harvard University in December 1989, Bennett called legalization proposals "morally scandalous," and he castigated those who thought "that the arguments in favor of drug legalization are rigorous, substantial, and

serious. They are not. They are, at bottom, a series of superficial and even disingenuous ideas that more sober minds recognize as a recipe for a public policy disaster." On the television program *This Week with David Brinkley,* he said legalization was "irresponsible nonsense."

Many proponents for reform referred to the alcohol model for

William F. Buckley, Jr. replies to William Bennett

William F. Buckley, Jr., editor of the conservative *National Review,* responded to William Bennett's approach to the drug war in his syndicated column:

> What if Bill Bennett should look at the problem hard in the face and conclude that prudent policy calls for licensing the sale of the drugs side-by-side with a massive national effort to warn against their consumption? If one were to remove from the price of drugs the overhead of sneaking it into the United States, killing or bribing all who stand in the way of this operation, and all who stand in the way of merchandising it in the streets, then the price of it would certainly collapse, and there would be no profit in its sale, save the modest profit of paying the licensed dispenser.

> Where some legalizers make a mistake is in suggesting that legalization might constitute a "solution" for the drug problem. That is careless, given that there is no solution to the drug problem. Conservative philosophy, by the way, rejects absolutely the use of the word "solution" except in narrow situations . . . What legalization advocates seek is a heavy mitigation of the concomitant consequences of the war on drugs: crime, the pre-emption of the energies of the justice system, and the engagement of society in a futile exercise. Legalization advocates are saying not that they have a solution to the drug problem, but that they are better off facing the situation that would eventuate after legalization than what they face today as drug warriors.

■■■

Milton Friedman Replies to William Bennett

In "An Open Letter to Bill Bennett" that appeared in the Wall Street Journal on 7 September 1989, Nobel Laureate economist Milton Friedman of Stanford University's Hoover Institute appealed as follows:

Dear Bill:

In Oliver Cromwell's eloquent words, "I beseech you, in the bowels of Christ, think it possible you may be mistaken" about the course you and President Bush urge us to adopt to fight drugs. The path you propose of more police, more jails, use of the military in foreign countries, harsh penalties for drug users, and a whole panoply of repressive measures can only make a bad situation worse. The drug war cannot be won by those tactics without undermining the human liberty and individual freedom that you and I cherish.

You are not mistaken in believing that drugs are a scourge that is devastating our society. You are not mistaken in believing that drugs are tearing asunder our social fabric, ruining the lives of many young people, and imposing heavy costs on some of the most disadvantaged among us. You are not mistaken in believing that the majority of the public share your concerns. In short, you are not mistaken in the end you seek to achieve.

Your mistake is failing to recognize that the very measures you favor are a major source of the evils you deplore. Of course the prob-

lem is demand, but it is not only demand, it is demand that must operate through repressed and illegal channels. Illegality creates obscene profits that finance the murderous tactics of the drug lords; illegality leads to the corruption of law enforcement officials; illegality monopolizes the efforts of honest law forces so that they are starved for resources to fight the simpler crimes of robbery, theft and assault. . . .

Had drugs been decriminalized 17 years ago, "crack" would never have been invented (it was invented because the high cost of illegal drugs made it profitable to provide a cheaper version) and there would today be far fewer addicts. The lives of thousands, perhaps hundreds of thousands of innocent victims would have been saved, and not only in the U.S. The ghettos of our major cities would not be drug-and crime-infested no-man's lands. Fewer people would be in jails, and fewer jails would have been built.

Columbia, Bolivia and Peru would not be suffering from narco-terror, and we would not be distorting our foreign policy because of narco-terror. Hell would not, in the words with which Billy Sunday welcomed Prohibition, "be forever for rent," but it would be a lot emptier.

Decriminalizing drugs is even more urgent now than in 1972, but we must recognize that the harm done in the interim cannot be wiped out, certainly not immediately. Post-

poning decriminalization will only make matters worse, and make the problem appear even more intractable. . . .

Alcohol and tobacco cause many more deaths in users than do drugs. Decriminalization would not prevent us from treating drugs as we now treat alcohol and tobacco: prohibiting sales of drugs to minors, outlawing the advertising of drugs and similar measures. Such measures could be enforced, while outright prohibition cannot be. Moreover, if even a small fraction of the money we now spend on trying to enforce drug prohibition were devoted to treatment and rehabilitation, in an atmosphere of compassion not punishment, the reduction in drug usage and in the harm done to the users could be dramatic.

This plea comes from the bottom of my heart. Every friend of freedom, and I know you are one, must be as revolted as I am by the prospect of turning the United States into an armed camp, by the vision of jails filled with casual drug users and of an army of enforcers empowered to invade the liberty of citizens on slight evidence. A country in which shooting down unidentified planes "on suspicion" can be seriously considered as a drug war tactic is not the kind of United States that either you or I want to hand on to future generations.

■■■

historical perspective. In a speech to the Drug Policy Foundation, U.S. District Judge Robert Sweet maintained that the U.S. policy of prison and prohibition has failed. He pointed out that profit from drugs was a main factor in street crime, and that decriminalizing marijuana would free up the justice system on a massive scale. He continued, "What we ought to do is try to get at the source of this problem, which is poverty and disillusionment, and put our resources behind that and turn it around. I suggest it is time to abolish the prohibition—to cease treating indulgence in mind-alteration as a crime. The result would be the elimination of the profit motive, the gangs, the drug dealers. Obviously, the model is the repeal of Prohibition and the end of Al Capone and Dutch Schultz."[48]

At a meeting of the U.S. Conference of Mayors on 25 April 1988 Baltimore's Mayor Kurt L. Schmoke and others also cited the failure of prohibition and called for a national debate on the legalization of drugs. Schmoke said in an inteview, "If we had invested in our public health system as much as we invested in our correction and criminal justice, we could control the drug problem to the point that it would not change the character of American cities. . . .

We can guarantee that if we continue doing what we're doing, we will fail. If we're going to have a new war on drugs, let it be led by the surgeon general, not the attorney general."[49]

Mayor Schmoke previously had been the chief prosecutor in Baltimore and had seen to the prosecution of thousands of drug cases, including a case in which his good friend Marcellus Ward, a police officer, was killed by drug dealers during a drug deal. Officer Ward had worn a tape recorder, and in prosecuting the case, Schmoke had to listen repeatedly to the tape. Later he wrote: "I didn't need to hear the sound of Marcellus Ward being shot to know that there was something terribly misguided about expecting law enforcement officers to stop drug abuse and drug trafficking.[50]

In *Legalize It? Debating American Drug Policy* Arnold Trebach threw himself into the debate, stating that, before the passsage of the Harrison Act in 1914,

Massive crime was not caused by wide drug availability. It is quite possible that prohibition was the leading cause of the huge increases in crime evident in the last 100 years. However, I do not attempt to make that argument here

---

■■■

No Praise for Folly

In a guest editorial for the *Washington Post* on 15 May 1988 Mayor Schmoke wrote:

Has the time come to add America's "war on drugs" to the long list of history's follies? In the view of historian Barbara Tuchman, to qualify as folly, a policy must not only be unsuccessful, it must be plainly against the interests of those in whose name it is being carried out. And folly has one more characteristic: Nobody wants to recognize it.

Whether the drug policies of the United States have reached the point of folly, I'm not prepared to say. But this much seems apparent: political maturity, intellectual honesty and justifiable concern about drug-related violence make raising the question long overdue.[51]

■■■

because so many other social and environmental factors—urbanization, economic dislocations, class conflicts, the breakdown of old family values and controls, to name only a few—have emerged over the last several decades that help explain crime . . . Nevertheless, I believe the data . . . seriously undercut the modern argument that legalizing drugs would certainly lead legions of citizens into lives of crime. . . . Virtually all of the data support my central thesis: the absence of national prohibition and the generally easy availability of drugs cannot be shown to have pushed significant numbers of people into crime. Under prohibition, crime rates have risen dramatically.

The mayors and police chiefs of the California cities of San Francisco, Oakland, and San Jose signed a resolution in May 1993 stating that:

The federal anti-drug effort, concentrating on police action and mandatory sentences, has in effect led to a race war, with disproportionate arrests of African Americans and Latinos. In addition, the multi-billion dollar War on Drugs campaign, started under the Nixon Administration in 1972, has proved so expensive that other services suffer.

The resolution was written by Milton Friedman and former San Jose police chief Joseph McNamara. They recommended "a new strategy focusing more on prevention and rehabilitation and less on arrests and punishment," and urged president Clinton and Congress "to convene a convention to recommend revisions of drug laws of the United States."[52]

In an effort to make peace, Senator Joseph Galiber introduced an act to establish a controlled substances law in the New York State Senate, calling for a Controlled Substance Authority to regulate the sale of all narcotics in much the same manner as the sale of alcohol. Drugs would be distributed by licensed physicians, pharmacists, clinics, and hospitals. The sales would be taxed, and prices and quality would be controlled. The containers would bear warning labels. Advertising would be restricted. The bill has been redrafted and reintroduced regularly since then, and stands as an exemplary alternative to the War on Drugs. Several other similar proposals are working their way through the legislatures of other states. The perennial California Marijuana Initiative, for example, concerns cannabis alone.

Despite pressure from media, analysts, and lobbies, President Bill

Clinton has chosen to ignore the concept of legalizing marijuana. White House press secretary Dee Dee Myers stated flatly in January 1994, "The president is against legalizing drugs, and he's not interested in studying the issue."[53] Thomas Constantine, the DEA figurehead under President Clinton, summed up the administration's ignorance on the subject: "I associate violent crime and drugs; they are totally intertwined in my mind. Many times people talk about the non-violent drug offender. That is a rare species. There is not some sterile drug type not involved in violence who is contributing some good to the community; that is ridiculous. They are contributing nothing but evil."[54]

DUTCH TREATMENT

The stance of the United States is by no means typical among world governments. For at least the last decade, a few nations have explored ways other than prohibition and punishment to manage cannabis. Holland, with its myriad hashish shops, practices a de facto legalization that works. Although the Dutch have prohibitive penal legislation against drug traffickers, the use of law enforcement is meant to reduce the supply of drugs, not to incarcerate upstanding citizens. "Prosecutional discretion" is used to pursue a more practical policy of tolerance toward the sale and possession of small quantities of cannabis.

The Dutch distinguish between cannabis, a "soft" drug, and "hard" synthetic drugs, such as heroin and amphetamines. They have been able to largely separate the two matters so that hashish smokers are not exposed to the temptations and dangers of stronger substances. Dutch drug policy emphasizes social control by means of adaptation and integration into society, rather than trying to enforce moral values by criminalizing and punishing drug users. Therefore, they attempt to reduce the demand for and the detrimental effects of drugs by educational and therapeutic means. The Dutch also consider nondrug social problems (poverty and the ghetto environment, racism, and access to social services) as a causal factor in substance abuse. The Dutch policy prevents users from being ostracized from society, alienated to a point where they cannot be reached and where the risks are extreme. Drug use is not encouraged, but users are given the opportunity to do so with full responsibility for protecting their health and with due respect for public safety.

■■■

On 28 April 1994, the highest court in Germany ruled that its citizens have the right to possess and consume small amounts of cannabis. Germany's sixteen states are currently agreeing on a uniform definition of personal use amounts.

On 5 May 1994, Columbia's high court legalized the personal possession and use of marijuana, hashish, and hallucinogens. The judges decided that the criminalization of personal possession of drugs was in violation of the citizens' constitutional right to "free development of the personality." The production, trafficking, and sale of drugs remains illegal.[55]

■■■

Simply by virtue of tolerating cannabis, Holland suffers much less from the problems associated with hard drugs than do other countries. Children are taught to cope with the risks of life, including drugs. As a result, the level of substance abuse among adolescents is much lower than in the United States and elsewhere. A recent study found that only 3 percent of Dutch teens smoke cannabis. The incidence of drug-related deaths also is very low. Locals and tourists enjoy hashish at liberty in public shops, where various forms of a notice in several languages tell customers: "No hard drugs. No aggression. No dealing in stolen goods. No entrance under the age of 16. In case of violation of these House Rules, the Police will be called immediately."[56]

In comparison, the U.S. Government, in its response to drugs, has imposed pretrial detention without bail, mandatory minimum prison sentences, and capital punishment for drug crimes, plus increased fines, forfeitures, asset seizures, and other gross transgressions of justice. American police use informants, undercover agents, entrapment and reverse stings, roadblocks, warrantless searches without probable cause, strip searches with compulsory urine and fecal samples, and drug-sniffing dogs, and they depend for more and more of their funds on bribes from hard-core smugglers. Civilians are obliged to undergo unreliable drug testing to gain and keep employment. The U.S. "war on drugs" is a fraudulent, institutionalized national psychosis that has cost Americans their civil rights, more than 150 billion tax dollars, and at least 100 million man-years spent in prisons. And the cost of this law enforcement includes countless deaths here and abroad.

The National Commission on Marihuana and Drug Abuse in 1972 foresaw and warned of these inevitable results even before Richard Nixon declared war on drugs:

Under certain conditions, perhaps, law enforcement alone might eliminate the illicit market in drugs. To achieve this, though, would require, at the least, multifold increases in manpower, a suspension of Fourth Amendment restraints on police searches, seizures, and wire-taps, wide-scale pretrial detention, abolition of the exclusionary rule and border controls so extreme that they would substantially hinder foreign commerce.[57]

Jamaican statesman Michael Manley criticized the harsh laws

against ganja in his country with logic that rings true for every country that is ostensibly democratic.

> When the issue is not crucial to the life of the society, yet the youngest offender, the smallest offender, must get a brutal, life-ruining penalty in the same way as the hardened and wicked offender, you are unfit to be legislators and unfit to be in charge of human beings, human lives in a civilized country.[58]

Hemp will continue to be woven into the tapestry of human life, and will continue to be controversial. Hopefully, in the future, when we step back and regard this tapestry, we will be able to see the thread stretching back into the most distant reaches of human past and forward into an unlimited future, with only the black mark in the second half of the twentieth century as a curiosity for the history books. The next few years promise to bring tumultuous change to the world of hemp; wouldn't it be wonderful if this change healed our democracy, too?

A HEMP UTOPIA

Every revolution has been driven by visions of a better tomorrow. Dreams of what-could-be founded this nation, and nothing is more traditionally American than to fight against the status quo. Here, then, is a vision of our hemp future worth fighting for. Probably not all aspects of this vision will come to pass, but they are all possible, today, with a few changes in infrastructure, law, and will. The year is 2020. We focus on the life of a North Carolina farmer. In honor of a famous citizen of that state, we'll call our farmer—Jesse.

Jesse rises, as usual, at dawn, leaving his wife and son still sleeping. He checks the temperature outside as he mixes up some ground hemp-seed hotcakes. Only 45° out! But it's still so warm inside; this Isohemp house keeps fooling him. He wonders if he'll have to use any heat at all this year. Maybe with the money he'll save on utilities he'll get some composite hempboard siding for the house, make it look just like his grandfather's old farmhouse that used to sit on the same ground when Jesse was a kid.

Jesse eats his hotcakes with syrup and strong black coffee. He used to have bacon with his breakfast every morning, but since the doctor told him about his high blood pressure he's turned vegetarian. It wasn't easy at first, but now that he eats hemp seed or hemp-seed oil a couple times a day his protein intake is up and his blood pressure is back to normal. Funny, it seems like he hasn't had a cold since then, either.

As he eats Jesse scans the morning paper—printed on recycled hemp and cereal straw, of course. There's more trouble with the OPEC nations. Their economies continue to collapse. No one will buy their oil, and other countries are trying to get them to pay for the pollution they are generating with their gas-powered vehicles, in accordance with the Pollution Summits of the previous decade. The United Nations wants to bring experts in to teach them to grow hemp in arid climates.

After breakfast Jesse pulls on his favorite hemp jeans—five years old, and still as tough as the day he got them—and goes out to the hemp fields. Some of the plants are sixteen feet tall now, slowly waving in the morning breeze. Their thick bark goes up almost to the tops of the plants, and there is hardly a flower in sight; this fiber-bred hemp has upped his yield 20 percent from what he used a few years ago. Jesse hops on his hemp-polymer tractor, filled with clean-burning hemp ethanol, and begins the process of harvesting. This part hasn't gotten much

easier since he started farming hemp at the turn of the century, but once it's down it goes straight to the decorticating plant that R. J. Morris converted from an empty prison. Jesse just gets the check from R. J. Morris, the same people who bought his tobacco from him when he used to farm it. Amazing how R. J. Morris fought so hard against the transition from tobacco to hemp, but then they were able to switch crops so easily and even introduce whole new clothing and paper lines. Jesse wonders if they are happy now that profits are up and they don't have the Surgeon General on their backs anymore.

Jesse is certainly happy. His son will have a working farm with healthy soil to inherit, and he saves money on pesticides and insecticides. Sure, it's more work to harvest hemp than tobacco, but the yield per acre is so much higher that he can farm fewer acres and make the same profit. He even donated some land to the Nature Conservancy last year, because it bordered on the Eastern Forest where the red wolves were coming back. That saved him some money on his taxes. Of course, his taxes were already low, since the economy is stronger and the law enforcement budget much smaller.

In the evening Jesse returns to the house. His son, back from third grade, is practicing tricks on his composite hemp skateboard. His wife is back from work—she's a technician at the biomass plant, converting waste from the hemp fields into electricity—and has already whipped up a batch of hemp-seed hummus for hors d'oeuvres. Jesse gets his bag of imported Grade A Hindu Kush *sativa* (the town coffee house was having a sale, so he treated himself) and rolls a cigarette. He used to have whiskey in the evening to unwind, but when he got an ulcer his doctor recommended hemp to clear it up. It worked like a charm, and Jesse found he didn't miss that deadening effect from alcohol.

The family is sitting down to dinner when a howl echoes across the fields. The red wolves! Jesse and his son head outside and climb up on the barn roof. A full moon is just rising out of the hemp field, and from the forest in the distance two, maybe three wolves are howling. Jesse remembers when the reintroduction pro-gram was started in the early '90s, but the wolves never did too well until the paper mills switched to hemp, the state stopped logging the eastern forest, and the wilder-ness came back. Now the white-tailed deer population is smaller and healthier, and the whole for-est seems more balanced.

Jesse's son says he just learned in American History how they used to shoot wolves on sight be-cause they thought they were evil. "That's true," says Jesse.

"But why would they do that?" asks his son. "Didn't they know wolves were a natural part of the forest?"

"People are scared of things they don't understand. Even things that make the world healthier and more beautiful."

"But that's just crazy," says his son. "That would be like . . . like if they made *hemp* illegal."

Jesse laughs, gazing around him at the fields rippling under the full moon. "Son, you're not going to believe the story I'm about to tell you."

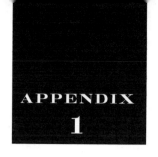

APPENDIX
1

THE HEMP
RESOURCE
GUIDE

Bookstores and Periodicals

Danger!
3968 St. Laurent Blvd., Montreal
Quebec HZW 1Y3 Canada
Phone: (514) 286-2998
Contact: Claude Lalumiere

Carries a full line of cannabis books and magazines.

Hemp BC
324 West Hastings
Vancouver, B.C. V6B 1K6 Canada
Phone: (604) 681-4620
Contact: Marc Emery

Offers a wide selection of grow guides, magazines, and books about cannabis.

Hemp World
P.O. Box 315
Sebastopol, CA 95473
Phone: (707) 887-7508
Fax: (707) 887-7639

EMAIL: hemplady@crl.com

Offers journals, books, and information as well as the publication *Hemp World: The International Hemp Journal.*

Hemptech
P.O. Box 820
Ojai, CA 93024-0820
Phone: (805) 646-HEMP
Contact: John W. Roulac

Offers the booklet *Industrial Hemp: Practical Products—Paper to Fabric to Cosmetics,* which reveals the many uses and benefits of the hemp plant for both the sociological and ecological arenas.

Hemp Times
111 E. 14th St., Suite 278
New York, NY 10003
Phone: (212) 505-1331
Fax: (212) 505-9021

A new quarterly celebrating the difference between hemp and marijuana through lifestyle and fashion features, how-to articles, and profiles of major hemp entrepreneurs. First issue June, 1996. Published by Trans-Hemp Company of America.

High Times
235 Park Ave. South, 5th floor
New York, NY 10003
Phone: (212) 387-0500

Publisher of a monthly magazine including hemp-related articles. Call (900) 988-8463, the *High Times* Hotline, for information on hemp-related issues.

Legal Marijuana/The Hemp Store
304 West Alabama
Houston, TX 77006
Phone: (713) 521-1134
Fax: (713) 528-HEMP
Contact: Richard Lee

Publisher of *Hemp Quarterly*, the publication that discusses hemp information, products, and people.

Longevity Book Arts
92470 River Rd.
Junction City, OR 97448
Phone: (503) 998-5710
Contact: Jonathan Root or Niya Nolting

Makers of tree-free and acid-free handmade hemp sketchbooks and journals.

Quick American Archives
1635 East 22nd Street
Oakland, CA 94060
Phone: (510) 535-0495
Fax: (510) 535-0437
Contact: Laura Shaw

Publisher of cannabis titles with a retail mail-order business.

Rainforest Botanical Laboratory
P.O. Box 1793
Gibsons, B.C. N0N 1V0 Canada

Offers the booklet *Nutritional and Medicinal Guide to Hemp Seed.*

Solar Age Press
Box 610
Peterstown, West Virginia 24963
Contact: Jack Frazier

Publisher of *Hemp Paper Report*, a bi-weekly hemp bulletin, and *Hemp Research Journal.*

Sweetlight Books
16625 Heitman Road
Cottonwood, CA 96022
Phone: (916) 529-5392
Contact: Guy Mount

Publisher of the quarterly magazine *Holy Smoke,* featuring spiritual and medical benefits of marijuana, hemp products, scientific research, legal concerns, illustrations, book reviews, poetry, organizational network news, advertising, and cannabis connections, as well as the novel *The Marijuana Mystery* and other hemp-related publications.

True Hemp Journal
P.O. Box 65130
St. Paul, MN 55165
Phone or fax: (612) 222-2628
Contact: John Birrenbach

A membership organization focusing on education and research. Publisher of the *True Hemp Journal.*

Weed World
P.O. Box 79
Rugby, Warwickshire CV23 8GR England
Phone: 0973 331121 (mobile)

Weed World is a quarterly publication that deals with all aspects of the use of cannabis and the legal issues concerning the plant.

E-Mail

David Borden of the Drug Reform Coordination Network
borden@eff.org

Cannabis Reform Coalition on the University of Massachusetts Amherst campus
verdant@twain.ucs.umass.edu

Electronic Frontier Foundation
barlow@eff.org

Marc Emery, publisher of Marijuana and Hemp Newsletter in Canada
marc_emery@mindlink.bc.ca

Exotic Gifts, a hemp importer and distributor
exotic@northcoast.com

Hemp BC, a retail store operating an on-line virtual store and information archives on the Internet at
http://www.hempbc.com.

Institute for Hemp is an educational and political center
instforhemp@delphi.com

Mari Kane, publisher of Hemp World Magazine
hemplady@crl.com

National headquarters for NORML
natlnorml@aol.com

President Clinton's office
president@whitehouse.gov

Vermont Hemporium office
vthemp@aol.com

Legalization, Advocacy, and Education

UNITED STATES

American Anti-Prohibition League
4017 SE Belmont St., Box 103
Portland, OR 97214
Phone: (503) 235-4524
Fax: (503) 235-1330
Contact: Floyd Ferris Landrath

A "political committee" registered with the Oregon Secretary of State's office, the league is retracing history, recreating the great "Anti-Prohibition Movement" of the early 1930s and applying it to today.

BACH (Business Alliance for Commerce in Hemp)
P.O. Box 71093
Los Angeles, CA 90071-0093
Phone: (310) 288-4152

BACH is an international business association that promotes hemp industries which research and produce information on hemp and advocates prompt legal reform.

CHA (Coalition for Hemp Awareness)
P.O. Box 9068
Chandler Heights, AZ 85227
Phone: (602) 988-9355
Fax:(602) 988-9438

The CHA functions as an informative network between groups and activists. CHA also presents a range of fine hemp products including clothing and accessories, bags, books, and navajo hemp weavings.

The Drug Policy Foundation
4455 Connecticut Ave., NW,
Suite B-500
Washington, DC 20008-2302
Phone: (202) 537-5005
Fax: (202) 537-3007
EMAIL dcondliffe@sorosny.org

The Drug Policy Foundation (DPF) is an independent, non-profit organization with 18,000 active members that researches and publicizes alternatives to current drug strategies. DPF believes that the drug war is not working and through a variety of programs the organization helps educate political leaders and the public about alternative drug control policies, which include harm reduction, decriminalization, medicalization, and legalization.

Hemp Industries Association (HIA)
P.O. Box 9068
Chandler Heights, AZ 85227
Phone: (602) 988-9355
Fax: (602) 988-9438

The pupose of the HIA is to represent the interests of the hemp industries and encourage the research and development of new hemp products.

Hemptech, Industrial Hemp Information Specialists
P.O. Box 820
Ojai, CA 93024
Phone: (805) 646-4367
Fax: (805) 646-7404
Contact: Angela Valley

Hemptech is a local network of communication and hemp experts working to reintroduce industrial hemp into the world economy. They publish books, reports, and offer other information services, including videos, to both individuals and organizations interested in the earth's premier renewable resource. The network is passionate about industrial hemp's role in improving both our economy and our environment and hopes to see bioregions throughout the world processing hemp in a sustainable manner.

Massachusetts Cannabis Reform Coalition
1 Homestead Road
Marblehead, MA 01945-1122
Phone: (617) 944-2266

A state affiliate of NORML

NORML
1001 Connecticut Ave., NW, Suite 1119
Washington, DC 20036
Phone: (900) 97-NORML or
        (202) 483-5500

The National Organization for the Reform of Marijuana Laws is a non-profit educational organization.

One Brown Mouse
P.O. Box 1794
Nederland, CO 80466
Phone: (303) 784-7122
Contact: Kathleen Chippi

Providers of information on any aspect of the re-legalization movement.

Vermont Grassroots
P.O. Box 537
Waitsfield, VT 05673
Phone: (802) 496-2387
Contact: Dennis Lane

An organization working toward an end to cannabis prohibition through literature, tours, and lectures.

CANADA

Canadian Hemp Association
312 Adelaide Street, West #608
Toronto, Ontario M5V-1R2 Canada
Phone: (416) 977-4159
Contact: Robin Ellis

An association of hemp textile farmers.

Crosstown Traffic
386 Richmond Rd.
Ottawa, Ontario K2A 0E8 Canada
Contact: Mike Foster

Devoted to decriminalization.

True North Hemp Company LTD
#103, 10324-WHYTE (82) Ave.
Edmonton, Alberta T6E-1Z8 Canada
Phone or fax: (403) 437-4367
Contact: Troy Stewart

The corporation supports and actively lobbies for the re-legalization of cannabis for medicinal and commercial use in Canada in order to promote economic growth in an environmentally sound and sustainable manner and to prevent the abuse of human rights.

EUROPE

Green Machine
Hoogte Kadijk 53-Bel Et.
1018 BE Amsterdam, the Netherlands
Phone: 31-20-638-1096
Fax: 31-20-638-2375

Green Machine is dedicated to the promotion of hemp products worldwide. They have helped to create the awareness that hemp is the world's premier renewable resource. Green Machine planted three hundred acres of hemp in England

with certified organic farmers. By growing hemp the farmers are able to work the land environmentally and profitably.

International Hemp Association (IHA)
postbus 75007
1070 AA Amsterdam, the Netherlands
Phone or fax: 31-20-618-8758

The IHA is a non-profit organization "Dedicated to the advancement of *Cannabis* through the dissemination of information." In light of the great economic potential of cannabis, the current legal restrictions hampering cannabis research and hemp cultivation should be considered. However, the IHA does not endorse a political stance on cannabis legislation, nor will it serve as a forum for the cannabis legalization debate.

Oesterreichisches Hanf-Institut
Duerergasse 3/4, A-1060
Wien, Austria
Phone: 00431-586-9429
Fax: 00431-586-9448
Contact: Mag. Helmuth Santler

The Austrian Hemp Institute is a non-profit organization with the aim of reintegrating hemp in the business world. The institute collects and provides information and publishes a quarterly magazine.

MUSEUMS AND LIBRARIES

The Hash Marihuana Hemp Museum
Oudezijds Achterburgwal 148
Amsterdam, the Netherlands
Phone or fax: 31-20-623-5961

Museo Civilito Contadina
Via S. Marina 35
40010 S. Marino di Bentivoglio
Bologna, Italy
Phone: 39-51-891050
Fax: 39-51-898377

RESEARCH

CARMEN Central Agricultural Raw Material Marketing and Development Network
Technologie Park
97222 Rimpar/Würzburg
Bavaria, Germany
Phone: 49-9365-80690
Fax: 49-9365-806955

Hemp Educational Research Board (HERB)
P.O. Box 7137
Boulder, CO 80306
Phone: (303) 225-8356

The purpose of HERB is to provide the technical support for the emerging industrial hemp industry. HERB will conduct research, develop hemp processing equipment, publish findings, participate in technical conferences, communicate with other researchers on the economic, environmental, energy, and other benefits of industrial hemp to provide the best possible information for policy makers, the agricultural community, business, financial and scientific communities, and the public.

Institut für Angewandte Forschung
Alteburgstrafse 150
72762 Reutlingen, Germany
Phone: 49-071-211536

Fax: 49-07121-211537
Contact: Martin Tubach

Engages in fiber separation research.

Manitoba Hemp Alliance
133 Albert St.
Winnipeg, Manitoba R3B 1G6 Canada
Phone: (204) 947-2315
Contact: Martin Moravcik

A non-profit group working to facilitate hemp research permits for Canadian farmers. The group has thus far imported six different types of hemp seed for agricultural research.

nova—Institute for Political and Ecological Innovation, Renewable Resources
Department, Thielstr. 35, 50354
Hürth, Germany
Phone or fax: 49-2233-72625
Contact: Michael Karus

Santa Monica office:
2324 30th St.
Santa Monica, CA 90405
Phone: (310) 392-8676
Fax: (310) 392-4105
Contact: Gero Leson

In its Renewable Resources Department, nova provides research, consulting, and coordinating services for the development of innovative and ecological processing technologies and products from renewable crops. The institute also develops socio-ecological concepts and conducts market potential and developmental studies.

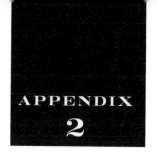

THE
HEMP
MARKETPLACE

Building Materials

C & S Specialty Builders
23005 N. Coburg Road
Harrisburg, OR 97446
Phone: (800) 728-9488

Offering quality hemp blended fiber-board and construction materials.

Canosmos
Ferme La Tuiliere 26560
Montfroc, France
Phone: 33-92-62-0074
Contact: Yves or Dominique Kühn

Developers of hemp-building materials and architecture.

Chènevotte Habitat
Le Verger F-72260
René, France
Phone: 33-43-97-4518
Fax: 33-43-97-6544
Contact: Mme. France Périer

Chènevotte Habitat offers environmentally safe hemp building materials and insulation. *Isochanvre* is nonflammable; forms a thermal and acoustical barrier with good thermic inertia; "breathes" to avoid condensation; is non-absorptive of water; is fungicidal, antibacterial, and waterproof; is inedible by rodents and termites; and is easy to use, supple, strong, and seven times lighter than concrete.

Clothing, Luggage, and Accessories

Anne's Custom Clothing
RR3
Blenheim, Ontario N0P 1A0 Canada
Phone: (519) 676-0930
Contact: Chris

Offers handmade hemp garments and accessories. Catalog available.

Hemp Out der Biorohstoff-shop
Ecke Weifsenburg und Schlosserstrafse
70180 Stuttgart, Germany
Phone: 49-711-640-4563

Producing the Marie Jane clothing line and devoted to using recycled and harmless material as well as educating the average person about hemp.

The Hemp Tribe
Van Oldenbarneveltstraat 126
3012 GW Rotterdam, the Netherlands
Phone: 31-10-413-3319
Fax: 31-10-412-6433
Contact: Argan or Linda Cos

Suppliers of fine hemp clothing.

Hempfully Yours
P.O. Box 923
Occidental, CA 95465
Phone: (707) 887-7741
Contact: Sarah Hutt or Beverly Tucker

A small cottage industry designing and making clothing and accessories.

Hemposphere
1540 S. Grand Ave. #A
Santa Ana, CA 92705
Phone: (800) 953-5562
Fax: (714) 953-6645
Contact: Dana Glazer

Hemposphere has debuted a line of Environmental Hemp backpacks and the line is available through catalogs and retail outlets. Environmental Hemp is a beautiful and functional accessory line of hats, bags, and wallets designed for the socially responsible individual.

Mindful Wear
20095 First Street West
Sonoma, CA 95476
Phone: (707) 939-9161
Contact: Max Salkin

Mindful Wear emphasizes environmentally friendly clothing, using organically grown fibers and natural dyes.

Planet Hemp
111 E. 14th St., Suite 279
New York, NY 10003
Phone: (212) 505-0101

A hemp-only retail store in New York City. Carries quality clothing, accessories, beauty products, and housewares by selected designers and manufacturers. Managed by the Trans-Hemp Company of America.

Terra Pax
1362 Pacific Ave. #213
Santa Cruz, CA 95060
Phone: (408) 459-8907
Fax: (408) 459-8914
Contact: James Cox

Carries high end, sustainably developed luggage.

Cosmetics and Body Care

Alma Rosa
Handelslei 12
2960 Brecht, Belgium
Phone: 03-281-43-93
Fax: 03-281-45-96
Contact: Jan Roelans

Offers Cannabliss hemp body-care products.

Artha
P.O. Box 20154
Oakland, CA 94620
Phone or fax: (510) 420-0696
Contact: Allysyn Kiplinger

Distributes handmade vegetarian hemp-seed-oil soaps.

Dupetit Natural Products
Haupstrafse 41
D-63930 Richelbach, Germany
Phone: 09378-367
Fax: 09378-394
Contact: Alfredo Dupetit

Offering cosmetics that are 100 percent natural and free from petrochemical and animal substances.

Hemp Garden Grofshandelsagentur
Olpenerstr. 242
51103 Köln, Germany
Phone or fax: 49-221-870-4767
Contact: Michael Mann

Distributor of hemp cosmetics.

Nektar
A-3300 Amstetten
Weberstrafse 6, Austria
Phone: 0-74-72-650-30
Fax: 0-74-72-650-304

Carries a complete cosmetic line based on natural hemp-seed oil.

SWIHTCO, the swiss hemp trading company
CH-3205 Mauss, Switzerland
Phone or fax: 41-31-751-30-05
Contact: Shirin Patterson

Sells hemp plants as insect repellent. Working toward using hemp in oil, cosmetics, and pharmaceuticals.

Food

Hempen Trail
28389 Big Basin Way
Boulder Creek, CA 95006
Phone: (408) 338-7113
Contact: Alan Brady

Producer of hemp seed ice cream and foods.

Hungry Bear Hemp Foods
P.O. Box 12175
Eugene, OR 97440
Phone: (503) 345-5216
Contact: Todd Dalotto

Producer of Vegan seedy treats.

Kind Distribution (formerly Deep See Ovens)
501 N. 36 Street #236
Seattle, WA 98103
Phone: (800) 436-7783
Fax: (206) 382-4080

Wholesaler and manufacturer of hemp goods including hemp seed treats, fabric, paper, oil, hemp rolling papers, and body care products.

Mama Indica's Hemp Seed Treats
Box 293
Ucluet, B.C. V0R 3A0 Canada
Phone: (604) 726-7239
Contact: Chris Bennett or Tracy
  Chester

Producer of yummy bars with sesame seeds, hemp seeds, nuts, honey, and brown sugar. These delicious treats are dry roasted to preserve the essential fatty acids.

Montana Hemp Traders
1455 Ft. MacLeod Trail
Eureka, MT 59917
Phone: (406) 889-3091
Contact: Jackie Beyer

Carrying a wide variety of hemp products including clothing, accessories, twine, books, videos, and treats.

The Ohio Hempery
7002 S.R. 329
Guysville, OH 45735
Phone: (800) BUY HEMP
Fax: (614)662-6446

Offers a wide selection of hemp products.

One Brown Mouse
P.O. Box 1794
Nederland, CO 80466
Phone: (303) 784-7122
Contact: Kathleen Chippi

Presently offering hemp cookie mix, hemp pancake mix, and packaged hemp cookies.

Sharon's Finest
P.O. Box 5020
Santa Rosa, CA 95402-5020
Phone: (707) 576-7050

Fax: (707) 545-7116
Contact: Rus Postel

The firm develops and markets unique new food products that meet certain dietary requirements, including fat-free, dairy-free, cholesterol-free, and meatless. HempRella is the first cheese alternative made from whole hemp seeds. Very high in essential fatty acids and GLA, low in fat. Also offers Hempeh Burgers.

Furnishings

Rising Star Futons
35 NW Bond Street
Bend, OR 97701
Phone: (800) 828-6711
Contact: Leslie Blok

Manufacturer and retailer of hemp futons.

Greener Pastures
526 Alder Lane
McKinleyville, CA 95521
Phone: (707) 839-8023
Contact: Laura Knight

Producer of hemp table linens.

Got It Covered
P.O. Box 14627
Santa Rosa, CA 95402
Phone: (707) 579-8443
Fax: (707) 829-5380
Contact: Joanne Walsh or Alan
  Silverman

Carriers of hemp table linens.

Media

Fotos
1726 Marvin Ave.
Los Angeles, CA 90019
Phone: (213) 937-3395
Contact: Jeff Eichen

Photographer of hempsters.

Hemp for Victory VHS videotape
HEMP (Help End Marijuana Prohibition)
5632 Van Nuys Blvd. #310
Van Nuys, CA 91401
Phone: (310) 392-1806

Marijuana's Greatest Hits Revisited
Compact disk, from Ichiban Records

Richard Fiorentino
7401 Neely Road
Guerneville, CA 95446
Phone: (707) 869-9773

Producer of hemp commercials.

She Who Remembers
Phone: (818) 287-8254

Offers audio/video material.

Phone: (800) 655-6944
Fax: (604) 370-1150
Contact: Odette Coleman

Outlet for hemp paper.

Living Tree Paper Co.
1430 Willamette St., Suite 367
Eugene, OR 97401
Phone: (800) 309-2974
    (503) 342-2974
Fax: (503) 687-7744
Contact: Carolyn Moran

Woman owned and operated, Living Tree Paper Co. is the maker of Tradition Bond™, an American-milled, tree-free hemp paper with 10% hemp, 10% Esparto grass, 60% agricultural by-products, and 20% post consumer waste.

Tree Free EcoPaper
121 S.W. Salmon, Suite 1100
Portland, OR 97215
Phone: (800) 775-0225
    (503) 295-6705
Fax: (503) 295-0883

Wholesaler and retailer of hemp paper and cover/card stock.

Paper

Alma Rosa
Handelslei 12
2960 Brecht, Belgium
Phone: 03-281-43-93
Fax: 03-281-45-96
Contact: Jan Roelans

Offers hemp paper.

EcoSource Paper
111-1841 Oak Bay Ave.
Victoria, B.C. V8R 1C4 Canada

Retailers: General

Alma Rosa
Handelslei 12
2960 Brecht, Belgium
Phone: 03-281-43-93
Fax: 03-281-45-96
Contact: Jan Roelans

Offers hemp paper and Cannabliss hemp body-care products.

American Hemp Mercantile
506 2nd Ave., Suite 1323
Seattle, WA 98104
Phone: (800) 469-4367
Fax: (206) 340-1086
Contact: Mary Donlan

Offers hemp fabric, clothing, and accessories as well as hemp books, treats, twine, and personal care items.

Cannabest
1536 Monterey Street
San Luis Obispo, CA 93433
Phone: (800) 277-0510
Contact: Lee Neel

The Cannabest mail-order catalog offers more than 150 hemp products from dozens of manufacturers. Printed in full color on hemp-based paper, the catalog presents the latest fashion accessories for men, women, and children as well as hemp seed and paper products, cloth, and more. Available for $3 (deductible from your first purchase).

Cannabis in Berlin Luckauer
Strasse 10
D-10969 Berlin, Germany
Phone: 49-30-615-6210
Fax: 49-30-264-4245
Contact: Stefan Thiele

Carries a large variety of hemp products and Hempstaff clothes. Also distributes wholesale seeds, cosmetics, books, fabrics, and clothes.

Crosstown Traffic
86 Richmond Rd.
Ottawa, Ontario K2A 0E8 Canada
Contact: Mike Foster

Provides a growing line of all things hempish.

Crucial Creations
550 S. 12th Ave., Suite 111
Tucson, AZ 85714
Phone: (602) 513-6615
Fax: (602) 746-0408
Contact: Denny Finneran

Offering 100 percent cannabis clothing and, in an effort to form alliances with other hemp companies to reintroduce Cannabis sativa for its many ecologically sustainable uses, Crucial Creations is now offering many other hemp products and brand names including Wise Up! Reaction Wear, Ohio Hempery, Headcase, American Hemp Mercantile, U. S. Hemp, and Odds & Ends.

Ecolution
2800 Juniper Street, Suite 2
Fairfax, VA 22031
Phone: (703) 207-9001
Fax: (703) 560-1175

Carrying a full line of hemp products including clothing, accessories, books, paper, and lip balm.

From All Over Imports
7-A 4120 Golfers Approach
Whistler, B.C. V0N 1B4 Canada
Phone: (604) 938-4959
Contact: Dave Currie

Growing selection of items related to cannabis.

Green Lands
P.O. Box 1651
1000 BR Amsterdam, the Netherlands
Phone: 31-20-627-1646
Fax: 31-20-627-3549
Contact: Erik Stofferis or Henk van
Dalen

Carriers of Hemp Eco products.

Green Machine
Hoogte Kadijk 53-Bel Et.
1018 BE Amsterdam, the Netherlands
Phone: 31-20-638-1096
Fax: 31-20-638-2375

Green Machine offers a full line of hemp products including clothing, fabric, paper, greeting cards, healthy Hempybars, organic seeds, oil, and massage and cosmetic oil.

Greener Alternatives
914 Mission St., Suite A
Santa Cruz, CA 95060
Phone: (408) 423-0701
Fax: (408) 423-0702
Contact: Robert Schwarz

An ecological hemp store featuring hemp clothing, fabric, body care products, seed oil, twine and rope, paper, books, accessories, and other green products.

Hemp BC
324 West Hastings
Vancouver, B.C. V6B 1K6 Canada
Phone: (604) 681-4620
Contact: Marc Emery

A retail store selling everything made of or about cannabis, including a full line of fabrics, seeds, clothing, oils, and ropes and twine as well as a full line of marijuana accessories including top-grade marijuana seeds, smoking equipment, grow guides and all magazines and books about cannabis. Hemp BC also operates an on-line virtual store and information archives on the Internet at http://www.hempbc.com.

Hemp Exchange
131 Albert St.
Winnipeg, Manitoba R3B 1G6 Canada

Phone: (204) 947-2315
Fax: (204) 956-5984
Contact: Martin Moravcik

A product information exchange office offering affordable hemp accessories.

Hemp Sacks
690 Nature Lane
Arcata, CA 95521
Phone: (707) 822-6972

Hemp hacky sacks are made entirely from the hemp plant. The outside is 100% Hungarian hemp twine. The inside is filled with 100% legal hemp seeds. Each sack is individually crafted and carries with it an attractive "Hemp facts" information tag printed on 100% post-consumer card stock. Their durability will give years of high kicking enjoyment.

House of Himalayan Hemp Traders
P.O. Box 4734
Kathmandu, Nepal
Fax: 977-1-472529

Legal Marijuana/The Hemp Store
1304 West Alabama
Houston, TX 77006
Phone: (713) 521-1134
Fax: (713) 528-HEMP
Contact: Richard Lee

Carries quality hemp products.

Montana Hemp Traders
1455 Ft. MacLeod Trail
Eureka, MT 59917
Phone: (406) 889-3091
Contact: Jackie Beyer

Carrying a wide variety of hemp products including clothing, accessories, twine, books, videos, and treats.

Of the Earth, Hemp and Organic Cotton Creations
916 W. Broadway, Suite 749
Vancouver, B.C. V5Z 1K7 Canada
Phone or fax: (604) 878-1268
Contact: Hélène Bisnaire or Richard Ziff

Offers infant, child, and adult clothing; bags, backpacks, and accessories. Using 100% hemp fabric or certified organically grown cotton fabric, all styles are offered in natural organic colors derived from renewable plant sources.

Off the Cuff
587 Johnson St.
Victoria, B.C. V8W 1M2 Canada
Phone: (604) 386-2221
Contact: Lisa Montroy

Retailers of hemp clothing, accessories, paper, yarn, seed, soap, and oils.

Original Sources
Box 7137
Boulder, CO 80306
Phone: (303) 225-8356

Offers an extensive line of hemp products and services including foods, fiber, fuel and oil, books and information, videos, consulting and analytical services, and seed.

Real Goods
966 Mazzoni Street
Ukiah, CA 95482-3471
Phone: (707) 468-9292
Fax: (707) 468-0301
Contact: Linda Malone

Real Goods is an environmental mail-order company that features a wide range of products for energy-efficient and earth-friendly living. The catalog regularly offers a variety of products made from hemp. For a free copy call (800) 762-7325.

Shakedown Street
276 King St.
W. Kitchener, Ontario N2G 1B7
Canada
Phone: (519) 570-0440
Contact: Bob Lazick or Derek Wildphong

Features rare books and magazines, smoking accessories, imported clothing, and Grateful Dead memorabilia.

Simply Better
90 Church Street
Burlington, VT 05401
Phone: (802) 658-7770
Contact: John Quinney

Carrier of fine hemp products including jewelry, hats, wallets, shoes, backpacks, fanny packs, vests, twine, and paper.

Still Eagle
557 Ward Street
Nelson, B.C. V1L 1T1 Canada
Phone: (604) 352-3844
Contact: Nick Smirnow

Offers food, fiber, medicine, paper, clothing, and more.

True Hemp North Company LTD
#103
10324-WHYTE (82) Ave.
Edmonton, Alberta T6E 1Z8 Canada
Phone or fax: (403) 437-4367
Contact: Troy Stewart

Carries a complete selection of hempen and informational products.

U.S. Hemp
461 W. Apache Trail #130
Apache Junction, AZ 85220
Phone: (800) 501-HEMP
(602) 983-7065

Retailers and wholesalers of books, clothing, accessories, and personal-care products. Mail-order catalog available.

Vermont Hemporium
Office: P.O. Box 65126
Burlington, VT 05406
Office phone: (802) 862-0225
Fax: (802) 865-2415
Store: 167 Lower Church Street
Burlington, VT 05401
Store phone: (802) 865-3088
Contact: Joe Shimek

Offers a broad array of hemp products.

What's the Alternative
9324 Main St.
Chilliwack, B.C. V2P 4M4 Canada
Phone: (604) 792-2442
Contact: Lynda Cabel

Carries all hemp products and related materials.

Textiles

Hemp Garden Grofshandelsagentur
Olpenerstr. 242
51103 Köln, Germany
Phone or fax: 49-221-870-4767
Contact: Michael Mann

Distributor of hemp textiles.

Hemp Textiles International
3200 30th Street
Bellingham, WA 98225
Orders: (800) 778-4367
Information: (360) 650-1684
Fax: (360) 650-0523
Contact: David Gould

An importer and wholesaler of fine cannabis hemp textile products.

Hemp Traders
2130 Colby Ave., Ste. #1
Los Angeles, CA 90025
Phone: (310) 914-9557
Fax: (310) 478-2108
EMAIL: hemptrader@aol.com

Carries the largest selection of hemp textiles.

Martin N. Youngberg Enterprises
5 Richard Court
Lincoln Park, NJ 07035

Engages in textile and analysis.

Owen Sercus A.A.P.
Textile and Marketing
Phone: (212) 924-7424
Fax: (212) 633-0807

Fashion Institute of Technology
Phone or fax: (212) 760-7593

U.S. Textile
404 West Pico Blvd.
Los Angeles, CA 90015
Phone: (213) 742-0840
Fax: (213) 742-0016
Contact: Simon Smiller

Offering Polish/Ukranian hemp fabric.

Wholesalers and Importers: General

American Hemp Mercantile
506 2nd Ave., Suite 1323
Seattle, WA 98104
Phone: (800) 469-4367
Fax: (206) 340-1086
Contact: Mary Donlan

Offers hemp fabric, clothing, and accessories as well as hemp books, treats, twine, and personal care items.

Aubout Company
1618 St. Lawrence Blvd.
Montreal, Quebec H2X 2T1 Canada
Phone: (514) 842-8595
Fax: (514) 843-8722
Contact: Larry Duprey

Distributor of hemp accessories, clothing, and twine.

Australian Hemp Products
227 Grinsell Street
Kotara, Newcastle N.S.W. 2289
Australia
Phone: 61-49-527802
Fax: 61-49-525211
EMAIL:
ouozhemp@cc.newcastle.edu.au
Contact: Grant Steggles

Offering quality hemp products.

Cannabis in Berlin
Luckauer, Strasse 10
D-10969 Berlin, Germany
Phone: 49-30-615-6210
Fax: 49-30-264-4245
Contact: Stefan Thiele

Carries a large variety of hemp products and Hempstaff clothes. Also distributes wholesale seeds, cosmetics, books, fabrics, and clothes.

Chicago Hemp Shop
1710 W. Fletcher, 2nd Floor
Chicago, IL 60657
Phone: (312) 472-5006
Contact: Mike Fink

Specializes in hemp teddy bears, clothing, and hats.

Crucial Creations
4550 S. 12th Ave., Suite 111
Tucson, AZ 85714
Phone: (602) 513-6615
Fax: (602) 746-0408
Contact: Denny Finneran

Offering 100 percent cannabis clothing and, in an effort to form alliances with other hemp companies to reintroduce Cannabis sativa for its many ecologically sustainable uses, Crucial Creations is now offering many other hemp products and brand names including Wise Up! Reaction Wear, Ohio Hempery, Headcase, American Hemp Mercantile, U. S. Hemp, and Odds & Ends.

Emperor's Clothing Co.
P.O. Box 2311
Winnipeg, Manitoba R3C 4A6 Canada
Phone: (204) 947-2315
Contact: Martin Moravcik

Asian and Canadian made hemp clothing, 100% hemp paper, hemp card stock, etc.

Hemp Garden Grofshandelsagentur
Olpenerstr. 242
51103 Köln, Germany
Phone or fax: 49-221-870-4767
Contact: Michael Mann

Distributor of hemp cosmetics, textiles, and paper.

Hemp Sacks
690 Nature Lane
Arcata, CA 95521
Phone: (707) 822-6972

Hemp hacky sacks are made entirely from the hemp plant. The outside is 100% Hungarian hemp twine. The inside is filled with 100% legal hemp seeds. Each sack is individually crafted and carries with it an attractive "Hemp facts" information tag printed on 100% post-consumer card stock. Their durability will give years of high kicking enjoyment.

Hemp Textiles International
3200 30th Street
Bellingham, WA 98225
Orders: (800) 778-4367
Information: (360) 650-1684
Fax: (360) 650-0523
Contact: David Gould

An importer and wholesaler of fine cannabis hemp textile products.

Hemp Traders
2130 Colby Ave., Suite 1
Los Angeles, CA 90025
Phone: (310) 914-9557
Fax: (310) 478-2108
EMAIL: hemptrader@aol.com

Carries the largest selection of hemp textiles.

The Hemp Tribe
Van Oldenbarneveltstraat 126
3012 GW Rotterdam, the Netherlands
Phone: 31-10-413-3319
Fax: 31-10-412-6433
Contact: Argan or Linda Cos

Suppliers of fine hemp clothing.

The Hempstead Company
2060 Placentia
Costa Mesa, CA 92627
Phone: (714) 650-8325
Fax: (714) 650-5853

Offers a variety of hemp products.

House of Himalayan Hemp Traders
P.O. Box 4734
Kathmandu, Nepal
Fax: 977-1-472529

Kind Distribution (formerly Deep See Ovens)
501 N. 36 Street #236
Seattle, WA 98103
Phone: (800) 436-7783
Fax: (206) 382-4080

Wholesaler and manufacturer of hemp goods including hemp-seed treats, fabric, paper, oil, hemp rolling papers, and body care products.

Legal Marijuana/The Hemp Store
1304 West Alabama
Houston, TX 77006
Phone: (713) 521-1134
Fax: (713) 528-HEMP
Contact: Richard Lee

Publisher of *Hemp Quarterly*, the publication that discusses hemp information, products, and people.

The Ohio Hempery
7002 S.R. 329
Guysville, OH 45735
Phone: (800) BUY HEMP
Fax: (614) 662-6446

Offers a wide selection of hemp products.

Steba Ltd.
1173 Budapest
Kaszáló u. 139, Hungary
Phone: 36-1-257-2745
Fax: 36-1-256-9802
Contact: Agnes Gyongyosi Palotas

A U.S./Hungarian joint venture formed to distribute hemp products traditionally produced in Hungary. The hemp products include twine, rope, cord, webbing in different sizes; sealing material for fittings; oil; fabric; hemp/leather combination items (backpacks, briefcases, folders, purses, etc.); hemp paper in different weights, and envelopes.

Still Eagle
557 Ward Street
Nelson, B.C. V1L 1T1 Canada
Phone: (604) 352-3844
Contact: Nick Smirnow

Offers food, fiber, medicine, paper, clothing, and more.

Two Star Dog
1526 62nd Street
Emeryville, CA 94608
Phone: (510) 655-4379
Fax: (510) 655-0209
Contact: Steven and Alan Boutrous

Makers of fine hemp clothing.

U.S. Hemp
461 W. Apache Trail #130
Apache Junction, AZ 85220
Phone: (800) 501-HEMP
     (602) 983-7065

Retailers and wholesalers of books, clothing, accessories, and personal-care products. Mail-order catalog available.

U.S. Textile
404 West Pico Blvd.
Los Angeles, CA 90015
Phone: (213) 742-0840
Fax: (213) 742-0016
Contact: Simon Smiller

Offering Polish/Ukranian hemp fabric.

Vermont Hemporium
Office: P.O. Box 9332
So. Burlington, VT 05407
Fax: (802) 865-2760
Store phone: (802) 865-3088
Contact: Joe Shimek, Lee Ann Schappe

Offers a broad array of hemp products.

NOTES

Notes to Introduction

1. Chris Conrad, *Hemp: Lifeline to the Future* (Los Angeles: Creative Xpressions Publishing, 1993), 130.

2. G. Hunsigi, *Outlook on Agriculture* 18, no. 3 (1989): 96–103.

Notes to Chapter 1

1. Andy Kerr, "Hemp to Save the Forests," *Wild Earth* (Summer 1994): 55.

2. Information on fiber crops is excerpted from the following sources: R. Bedetti and N. Ciaralli, *Cellulosa e Carta* 26 (1976): 27–30; J. Berger, *The World's Major Fibre Crops: Their Cultivation and Manuring* (Zurich: Centre D'Etude De L'Azote, 1969); A. Bosia, *Cellulosa e Carta* 26 (1976): 32–36; B. R. Christie, *CRC Handbook of Plant Science in Agriculture*, vol. 2 (Boca Raton, Fla.: CRC Press, 1987), 71–85; Paul Hawken, *The Ecology of Commerce* (New York: HarperCollins, 1993), 149; R. H. Kirby, *Vegetable Fibres: Botany, Cultivation, and Utilization* (New York: Interscience Publishers, 1963); J. W. Purseglove, *Tropical Crops: Dicotyledons* (New York: John Wiley and Sons, 1966), 40–44; David W. Walker, "Can Hemp Save Our Planet?" NORML 20th Annual Conference (30 August–2 September 1990), reprinted in *Hemp Line* 1, no. 1 (1992): 18–20, and 1, no. 2 (1992): 14–18; C. J. West, *Paper Trade Journal* (13 October 1921): 46, 48.

3. Hawken, *The Ecology of Commerce,* 3, 22, 29.

4. West, *Paper Trade Journal,* 46, 48.

5. Hawken, *The Ecology of Commerce,* 40–44.

6. Mitch Lansky, *Beyond the Beauty Strip* (Gardiner, Maine: Tilbury House, 1992), 252, 257.

7. Proceedings, Bioresource Hemp Symposium (March 1994), Frankfurt, Germany.

8. Information on fiber crops from: Anne L. Ash, *Economic Botany* 2 (1948): 158–169; D. Catling and J. Grayson, *Identification of Vegetable Fibres* (London: Chapman & Hall, 1982), 71–78; W. Hoffman, "Hanf, Cannabis sativa," *Handbuch der Pflanzenzuchtung,* part 5 (Hamburg: Paul Parey), 204–263; B.C. Kundu, Indian *Botanical Society Journal* 21 (1942): 93–128.

9. Integrated Biofuels Research Program, Phase II Final Report, Hawaii Natural Energy Institute, Hawaii, August 1990.

10. Conrad, *Hemp: Lifeline to the Future,* 103–114.

11. Haney and Kutscheid, *American Midland Naturalist* 93, no. 1 (January 1975): 1–24.

12. Lynn Osburn, *Energy Farming in America* (Frazier Park, Calif.: Access Unlimited, 1992).

13. Agua Das, Box 7137, Boulder, Colo. 80306, 303-225-8356.

14. Ed Rosenthal, *HempToday* (Oakland, Calif.: Quick American Archives), 139–143.

15. Stanley Manahan, *Energy from Photosynthesis,* 3rd ed. (Columbia, Mo.: University of Missouri Press), 439.

16. 2425 Eighteenth St. NW, Washington, DC 20009-2096, 202-232-4108.

17. Jack Herer, *Hemp and the Marijuana Conspiracy: The Emperor Wears No Clothes* (Van Nuys, Calif.: HEMP Publishing, 1994).

18. Sackett and Hobbes, *Hemp: A War Crop* (New York: Mason & Hanger, 1942).

19. Lyster Dewey, "Hemp," *USDA Yearbook* (Washington, DC: U.S. Government Printing Office, 1913).

20. T. Malyon and A. Henman, *New Scientist* (13 November 1980): 433–435.

21. *Toronto Globe and Mail* (15 June 1994), A25; *Toronto Globe and Mail* (7 June 1994), A1, A4.

22. B. B. Robinson, "Hemp," *USDA Farmers' Bulletin No. 1935* (Washington, DC: U.S. Government Printing Office, 1943); *The Humorous Hemp Primer,* (Berlin, 1943) reprinted in *The Emperor Wears No Clothes.*

23. John W. Roulac, ed., *Industrial Hemp: Practical Products—Paper to Fabric to Cosmetics* (Ojai, Calif.: Hemptech, 1995).

24. B. R. Lazarenko and J.B. Gorbatovskaya, *Applied Electrical Phenomena* 6 (March–April, 1966).

25. Herer, *The Emperor Wears No Clothes,* 104–111; and Don Wirtshafter, *The Schlichten Papers* (Guysville, Ohio: The Ohio Hempery, 1994).

26. Proceedings, Bioresource Hemp Symposium (March 1994).

Notes to Chapter 2

1. Dan Bensky and Andrew Gamble, *Chinese Herbal Medicine: Materia*

Medica (Seattle: Eastland Press, Inc., 1993).

2. Sources: N. P. Manandhar, *Economic Botany* 45 (1991): 63; P. Francis, *Economic Botany* 38 (1984): 197–200; Uday Chang and G. King, *The Materia Medica of the Hindus* (n.p.: Thacker, Spink & Co., 1877); Lise Manniche, *An Ancient Egyptian Herbal* (Austin: University of Texas Press, 1989); and Francois Rabelais, *Gargantua and Pantagruel,* trans. Burton Raffel (New York: W. W. Norton & Co., 1990).

3. William B. O'Shaughnessy, *Trans. Med. and Physical Soc. Bengal* 8 (1838–1840): 421–469.

4. Sources: L. Aubert-Roche, *Documents and Observations Concerning the Pestilence of Typhus* (Paris: J. Rouvier, 1843); J. R. Rodger, *J.A.M.A.* 217, no. 12 (1971): 1705–1706; J. Shaw, *Madras Q. Med. J.* 5 (1843): 74–80; and R. Inglis, *Medical Times* 12 (1854): 454.

5. V. Robinson, *Medical Review of Reviews* 18 (1912): 159–169.

6. L. Grinspoon and J. B. Bakalar, *J.A.M.A.* 273 (1995): 1875–1876.

7. M. E. West, *Nature* 351 (27 June 1991): 703–704; and M. E. West and A. B. Lockhart, *West Indies Med. J.* 27 (1978): 16–25.

8. Keith Green, "Marijuana Effects on Intraocular Pressure," in *Glaucoma: Applied Pharmacology of Medical Treatment,* ed. Stephen M. Drance and Arthur H. Neufeld (Grune & Stratton, 1984), 507–526; K. Green et al., *Exper. Eye Res.* 23 (1976): 443–448; 24 (1977): 189–196; 27 (1978): 239–246.

9. R. S. Hepler and I. M. Frank, *J.A.M.A.* 217(1971): 1392; W. W. Dawson et al., *Investig. Opthalmol.* 16, no. 8 (1977): 689–699; and H. Mohan and G. C. Sood, *Brit. J. Opthalmology* 48 (1964): 160.

10. Sources for the discussion of cannabis as an anti-emetic include: S. E. Sallan et al., *New Engl. J. Med.* 293 (1975): 795–797; S. E. Sallan et al., *New Engl. J. Med.* 302 (1980): 135–138; L. E. Orr et al., *Arch. Int. Med.* 140 (1980): 1431–1433; R. J. Gralla et al., *Proc. Amer. Soc. Clin. Oncol.* 1 (1982): 58; E. A. Formukong et al., *Phytotherapy Res.* 3, no. 6 (1989): 219–231.

11. M. Kleiman and R. Doblin, *Annals of Internal Medicine* (1 May 1991).

12. W. D. Lyman et al., *J. Neuroimmunology* 23 (1989): 73–81; R. Karler et al., *Life Sci.* 15 (1974): 9131–9147.

13. *Ther. Gazz.* 11 (1887): 4–7, 124.

14. L. Vachon et al., *Chest* 70, no. 3 (1976): 444.

15. D. P. Tashkin et al., *Amer. Rev. Respir. Dis.* 109 (1974): 420–428; 122 (1975): 377–386.

16. R. Gordon et al., *Eur. J. Pharmacol.* 35 (1976): 309–313.

17. Other sources for discussion of the effect of cannabis on breathing include: J. Hartley et al., *British Journal of Clinical Pharmacology* 5, no. 6 (1978): 523–525; and J. Sirek, "Importance of Hemp Seed in TB Therapy" (in Czech), *Acta*

Univ. Palack. Olomuc. 6 (1955): 93–108.

18. J. R. Reynolds, *The Lancet* 1 (22 March 1890): 637–638; and J. M. Cunha et al., *Pharmacology* 21 (1980): 175–185.

19. W. A. Check, *J.A.M.A.* 241, no. 23 (1979): 2476.

20. P. Consroe et al., *Intl. J. Neuroscience* 30 (1982): 277–282; and G. Giusti et al., *Experientia* 33 (1977): 257; M. Gildea and W. Bourne, *Life Science* 10 (1977): 133–140.

21. L. S. Harris et al., "Anti-tumor properties of cannabinoids," in Monique C. Braude and Stephen I. Szara, *Pharmacology of Marihuana* (New York: Raven Press, 1976); and L. S. Harris, *Pharmacologist* 16 (1974): 259.

22. A. C. White et al., *J. Natl. Cancer Inst.* 56 (1976): 655–658; and M. A. Friedma, *Cancer Biochem. Biophysics* 2, no. 2 (1977): 51–54.

23. J. Kabelik et al., *Bull. Narc.* 12 (1960): 5–23.

24. Z. Krejci, *Pharm. Indust.* 13 (1958): 155–157; Z. Krejci, *Pharmazie* 12 (1957): 439–443; 14 (1959): 279–281; and B. van Klingerin and M. ten Ham, *Antonie van Leeuwenhoek* 42 (1976): 9–12.

25. Toronto *Globe & Mail* (16 June 1994), 20.

26. Jacques-Joseph Moreau, *Hashish and Mental Illness* (New York: Raven Press, 1973); A. Brigham, *American Journal of Insanity* 2 (1846): 275–281.

27. G. T. Stockings, *J. Mental Sci.* 90 (1944): 772.

28. J. J. Moreau, Lancette *Gazette Hopital* 30 (1857): 391; W. Regelson et al., "THC As an Effective Anti-depressant," in *Pharmacology of Marihuana,* ed. Monique C. Braude and Stephen I. Szara, vol. 2, 777; and J. Kotin et al., *Arch. Gen. Psychiatr.* 28 (1973): 345–348.

29. R. K. Turner et al., *Arch. Int. Pharmacodyn. Ther.* 214, no. 2 (1975): 254–262.

30. S. S. Mishra and I. Sahai, *7th Intl. Congress of Pharmacology* (Paris, 16–21 July 1978), 168.

31. D. S. Kosersky et al., *Eur. J. Pharmacol.* 24 (1973): 1–7.

32. E. A. Formukong et al., *Inflammation* 12 (1988): 361–371.

33. B. Carty et al., U.S. Patent 4,917,889 (Cl. 424/693.1), 17 April 1990.

34. S. L. Milstein, *Intl. J. Pharmacopsychiat.* 10 (1975): 177–182; S. Y. Hill, *J. Pharmacol. Exper. Ther.* 188 (1974): 415–418; and R. Noyes et al., *J. Clin. Pharmacol.* 15 (1975): 139–143.

35. J. W. Fairbairn and J. T. Pickens, *Brit. J. Pharmacology* 69 (1980): 491–493.

36. J. M. Barrett et al., *Biochem. Pharmacol.* 34 (1985): 2019–2024.

37. Newsbank (1991): HEALTH 93: G10.

38. L. J. Thompson and R. C. Proctor, "Pyrahexyl in the Treatment of Alcoholic and Drug Withdrawal Conditions," in *The Marihuana Papers,* ed. David Solomon (New York: Bobbs-Merrill Co., Inc., 1966), 380–387.

39. C. M. Rosenburg, *Psychopharmacol. Bull.* 9 (1973): 25; J. Scher, *Amer. J. Psychiatry* 127 (1971): 971–972; and J. B. Mattison, *St. Louis Med. Surg. J.* 61 (1891): 265–271.

40. E. Birch, *Lancet* 1 (1889): 625.

41. J. B. Mattison, *Can. Med. Rec.* 13 (1885): 73–84.

42. J. B. Mattison, *St. Louis Med. Surg. J.* 61 (1891): 266; S. Allentuck and K. M. Bowman, *Amer. J. Psychiatry* 99 (1942): 250.

43. E. A. Carlini and J. M. Cunha, *J. Clin. Pharmacol.* 21, Suppl. (1981): 417–427.

44. P. S. Morahan et al., *Infect. Immunology* 23, no. 3 (1979): 670–674.

45. G. Lancz et al., *Proc. Soc. Exper. Biol. & Med.* 196 (1991): 401–404.

46. H. A. Hare, *Ther. Gazz.* 11 (1887): 225.

47. J. J. Reynolds, *Lancet* 1 (1890): 637.

48. J. Zias et al., *Nature* 316 (20 May 1993): 215; and P. Prioreschi and D. Babin, *Nature* 364 (19 August 1993): 680.

49. J. B. Mattison, *St. Louis Med. Surg. J.* 61 (1891): 266.

50. William Osler, *The Principles and Practice of Medicine,* 8th ed. (New York: n.p., 1913), 1089; Z. Volfe et al., *Intl. J. Clin. & Pharmacol. Res.* 5 (1985): 243–246.

51. J. S. Jones, *Lancet* (1978): 1053; and G. See, *Ther. Gazz.* 14 (1890): 684–685; *J.A.M.A.* 15 (1890): 540; and *Lancet* 2 (1890): 631–632.

52. J. Grigor, *Monthly J. Med. Sci.* 15 (1852): 124–125.

53. J. Brown, *Brit. Med. J.* 1 (26 May 1883): 1002.

54. R. Batho, *Brit. Med. J.* 1 (26 May 1883): 1002.

55. Lynn Osburn, *Hemp Line Journal* 1, no. 2 (1992): 12, 13, 21; H. B. Vickery et al., *Science* 92 (4 October 1940): 317–318; *The Wealth of India: Raw Materials,* vol. 2 (Delhi: Council of Scientific and Industrial Research, 1950), 58–64.

56. M. Shinogi and I. Mori, *Yakugaku Zasshi* 98, no. 5 (1978): 569–576; Harry A. Waisman and C. A. Elvehjem, *J. Nutrition* 16, no. 2 (August 1938): 103–114; and Rosenthal, *HempToday.*

57. T. B. Osborne, *Amer. Chem. J.* 14 (1892): 662; and *J.A.C.S.* 21 (1899): 486 and 24 (1902): 28, 39; T. B. Osborne and L. B. Mendel, *J. Biol Chem.* 13 (1912): 233.

58. A. J. St. Angelo et al., *Arch. Biochem. and Biophysics* 124 (1968): 199–205.

59. Conrad, *Lifeline to the Future,* 143.

60. A. Kemmoku et al., *Bull. Faculty of Education, Utsonomiya University* 42, no. 2 (1992): 165–172.

61. *Herbal Pharmacology in the People's Republic of China* (Washington, DC: National Academy of Sciences, 1975), 111; A. Weil, *Natural Health Magazine* (March–April 1993): 10–12.

62. J. C. Hammond, *Poultry Science* 23, no. 1 (1944): 78; A. H. Folger, "The Digestibility of Perilla Meal, Hemp Seed Meal, and Babassu Meal, as Determined for Ruminants," *University of Califor-*

nia (Berkeley) College of Agriculture Bulletin #604 (January 1937); and H. C. Mookerjee, *Modern Review* 84 (1948): 447.

63. U. Erasmus, *Fats That Heal, Fats That Kill* (Burnaby, British Columbia: Alive Books, 1993), 287–292.

64. Lester Grinspoon, *Marihuana Reconsidered* (Oakland, Calif.: Quick American Archives, 1994), X.

65. *Report of the Indian Hemp Drugs Commission (1893–1894),* 8 vols. (Simla, India: British Government Central Printing House, 1894).

66. Tod Mikuriya, *International J. of the Addictions* (Spring, 1968); and John Kaplan, *Report of the Indian Hemp Drugs Commission: Summary Volume* (Silver Springs, Md.: Jefferson Press, 1969).

67. Siler Committee, *Canal Zone Papers* (Washington, DC: U.S. Government Printing Office, 1931).

68. Ibid.

69. New York Mayor's Committee on Marihuana, *The Marihuana Problem in the City of New York* (Metuchen, N.J.: Scarecrow Reprint Corp., 1973).

70. Hallucinogens Subcommittee of the British Advisory Committee on Drug Dependence, The *Wooton Report on Cannabis* (Her Majesty's Stationery Office, 1968); and *Nature* 221 (1969): 205–206.

71. National Commission on Marihuana and Drug Abuse, *Cannabis: Signal of Misunderstanding* (Washington, DC: U.S. Government Printing Office, 1972).

72. Vera Rubin and Lambros Comitas,

Ganja in Jamaica: A Medical Anthropological Study of Chronic Marihuana Use (The Hague: Mouton, 1975); and G. G. Nahas, *Bulletin on Narcotics* 37, no. 4 (1985): 15–29.

73. Rubin and Comitas, 1975.

74. Ibid.

75. Melanie C. Dreher, *Working Men and Ganja* (Philadelphia, Penn.: Institute for the Study of Human Issues, 1982).

76. W. E. Carter and P. L. Doughty, *Annals N.Y. Acad. Sci.* 282 (1976): 2–16.

77. J. M. Fletcher et al., *Contemporary Drug Problems* 7, no. 1 (1978): 3–34; P. Satz et al., *Ann. N.Y. Acad. Sci.* 282 (1976): 266–306; and W. Carter, ed., *Cannabis in Costa Rica: A Study in Chronic Marijuana Use* (Philadelphia, Penn.: Institute for the Study of Man, 1980).

78. C. N. Stefanis and M. R. Issodorides, Science 191, no. 4233 (1976): 1217; C. Stefanis et al., *Hashish! A Study of Long-Term Use* (New York: Raven Press, 1977); J. C. Bouloulgouris et al., *Annals N.Y. Acad. Sci.* 282 (1976): 17–23; and R. L. Dornbush and A. Kokkevi, *Annals N.Y. Acad. Sci.* 282 (1976): 58–63, 313–322.

79. NewsBank (1983): LAW 67: E14.

80. Grinspoon, *Marijuana Reconsidered,* X.

81. Advisory Council on the Misuse of Drugs, *Report of the Expert Group on the Effects of Cannabis Use* (United Kingdom Home Office, 1982).

82. D. P. Tennant et al., *J.A.M.A.* 216

(1971): 1965–1969; C. Zwillich et al., *J. Clin. Res.* 25, no. 2 (1977): 136-A; W. R. McConnel et al., *Fed. Proc.* 34, no. 3 (1975): 782.

83. G. L. Huber et al., *Chest* 77 (1980): 403–410; C. Leuchtenberger et al., *Nature* 241 (1973): 137–139.

84. R. Charles et al., *Clinical Toxicology* 14, no. 4 (1979): 433–438; and T. E. Piemme, *N. Engl. J. Med.* 285, no. 2 (1971): 124.

85. J. M. Hanna et al., *Aviation, Space and Environ. Med.* 47 (1976): 634–639; I. E. Waskow et al., *Arch. Gen. Psychiatry* 22 (1970): 97–107; and E. L. Abel, *Experientia* 29, no. 12 (1973): 1528–1529.

86. G. F. Ewens, *Insanity in India, Its Symptoms and Diagnosis with Reference to the Relation of Crime and Insanity* (Calcutta: n.p., 1908); A. Heyndrickx et al., *J. Pharm. Belg.* 24 (1969): 375; *Chem. Abstracts* 72 (1970): 41177t; and N. E. Gary and V. Keylon, *J.A.M.A.* 211, no. 3 (1970): 501.

87. J. C. Garriott *N. Engl. J. Med.* 285 (1971): 86–87; and *Chem. Abstracts* 74 (1971): 97268g.

88. S. Burnstein et al., *Molecular Pharmacology* 15, no. 3 (1979): 633–640.

89. R. C. Kolodny et al., *N. Engl. J. Med.* 290 (1974): 872–874; J. H. Mendelson et al., *N. Engl. J. Med.* 291 (1974): 1051–1055; J. W. Coggins et al., *Ann. N.Y. Acad. Sci.* 282 (1976): 148–161; and W. C. Hembree et al., "Changes in Human Spermatazoa Associated with High-Dose Marihuna Smoking,"

in *Marihuana: Biological Effects,* ed. G. G. Nahas and W. D. M. Paton (Oxford: Pergamon Press, 1979), 429–439.

90. M. C. Dreher, K. Nugent, and R. Hudgins, "Prenatal Marijuana Exposure and Neonatal Outcomes in Jamaica: An Ethnographic Study," *Pediatrics* 93, no. 2 (1994): 254–260.

91. J. Harmon and M. A. Aliapoulios, *N. Engl. J. Med.* 287 (1975): 936; J. Harmon and M. A. Aliapoulios, *Surg. Forum* 25 (1974): 423–425; W. Cates and J. Pope, *Amer. J. Surgery* 134 (November 1977): 613–615; and C. Pere-Vitoria, *Rev. Iber. Endocrinol.* 23, no. 137 (1976): 437–44.

92. *Brit. Med. J.* 1 (1969): 797.

93. J. Buckley, "A Case Study of Acute Nonlymphoblastic Leukemia—Evidence for an Association with Marihuana Exposure," in *Cannabis: Physiology, Epidemiology, Detection,* ed. G. Nahas and C. Latour (Boca Raton, Fla.: CRC Press, 1993), 155; and H. Tuchmann-Duplessis, "Effects of Cannabis on Reproduction," in *Cannabis: Physiology, Epidemiology, Detection,* ed. G. Nahas and C. Latour, 187–193.

94. R. G. Heath et al., *Biol. Psychiatry* 15 (1980): 657–690; J. W. Harper et al., *Neurosci. Res.* 3 (1977): 87–93; and A. Campbell et al., *Lancet* 2 (1971): 1219–1225.

95. Grinspoon, *Marijuana Reconsidered,* 387.

96. Arnold Relman, ed., *Marijuana and Health* (Washington, DC: National Academy Press, 1982).

97. A. N. Chowdhury and N. K. Bera, *Addiction* 89 (1994): 1017–1020.

98. Charles Tart, *On Being Stoned* (Palo Alto, Calif.: Science and Behavior Books, 1971); L. D. Clark et al., *Arch. Gen. Psychiatry* 23 (1970): 193–198; L. Vachon et al., *Psychopharmacologia* 39 (1974): 1–11; J. R. Tinklenberg, *Psychopharmacology* 49 (1976): 275–279; W. D. M. Paton and June Crown, eds., *Cannabis and Its Derivatives* (London: Oxford University Press, 1972); and Andrew Weil, *The Natural Mind* (Boston: Houghton Mifflin Co., 1972), 96–97.

99. D. J. Spencer, *Brit. J. Addiction* 65 (1970): 369–372; D. S. Chopra and J. W. Smith, A*rch. Gen. Psychiatry* 30 (1974): 24–27; J. A. Talbott and J. W. Teague, *J.A.M.A.* 210 (1969): 299–302; F.S. Tennant, *J.A.M.A.* 221 (1972): 1146–1149; and D. A. Treffert, *Amer. J. Psychiatry* 135 (1978): 1213–1215.

100. C. F. Darley et al., *Psychopharmacologia* 29 (1973): 231–238; 37 (1974): 139–149; E. L. Abel, *Nature* 227 (1970): 1151–1152; 231 (1971): 260–261; and Kenton Robinson, "Synapse relapse? It's not your druggie past," *Las Vegas Review Journal* (13 November 1994): 10-J.

101. Robert Berkow, ed., *Merck Manual of Diagnosis and Therapy* (Rahway, N.J.: Merck Sharp & Dohme Research Laboratories, 1987).

102. J. Shedler and J. Block, *Amer. Psychologist* 45 (May 1990): 612–630.

103. NewsBank XXV (1994): LAW 9: C3.

104. N. Zinberg and A. Weil, *Nature* 226 (1970): 119.

105. H. Kolansky and W. Moore, *J.A.M.A.* 216 (1971): 486–492.

106. Grinspoon, *Marijuana Reconsidered,* XX.

107. Rubin and Comitas, *Ganja in Jamaica,* 1975.

108. E. J. Corey et al., *J. Amer. Chem. Soc.* 106 (1984): 1503–1504.

109. *Science News* 134 (26 Nov. 1984): 350.

110. Kathy A. Fackelman, *Science News* 143 (6 February 1993): 88–89, 94; Sean Munro et al., *Nature* 365 (2 September 1993): 61–65; and L. Matsuda et al., *Nature* 346 (9 August 1990): 561–564.

111. W. A. Devane, *Trends Pharmacol. Sci.* 15, no. 2 (1994): 40–41.

Notes to Chapter 3

1. Terence McKenna, "Plan, Plant, Planet," *Whole Earth Review* (Fall 1989): 6.

2. Carl Sagan, *The Dragons of Eden* (New York: Random House, 1977), 191.

3. Richard Evans Schultes and Albert Hofmann, *Plants of the Gods* (Rochester, Vt.: Healing Arts Press, 1992), 95.

4. Ernest L. Abel, *Marijuana: the First Twelve Thousand Years* (New York: Plenum Press, 1980), 19.

5. Mircea Eliade, *Shamanism* (New York: Pantheon Books, 1973).

6. Edward M. Brecher and the editors of *Consumer Reports: Licit and Illicit Drugs* (Boston: Little Brown, 1972), 398.

7. C. Creighton, "On Indications of the Hasheesh Vice in the Old Testament," *Janus* 8 (1903).

8. Gabriel G. Nahas, *Marihuana: Deceptive Weed* (New York: Raven Press, 1973), 3.

9. Chris Bennett, Lynn Osburn, and Judy Osburn, *Green Gold, the Tree of Life: Marijuana in Magic and Religion* (Frazier Park, Calif.: Access Unlimited, 1995), 193.

10. Grinspoon, *Marihuana Reconsidered*, 58–59.

11. A. Symons, trans., *Baudelaire: Prose and Poetry* (New York: Albert and Charles Boni, 1926), 275.

12. Brecher, *Licit and Illicit Drugs*, 408.

13. G. W. Grover, *Shadows Lifted or Sunshine Restored on the Horizon of Human Lives: A Treatise on the Morphine, Opium, Cocaine, Chloral, and Hashish Habit* (Chicago: Stronberg, Allen & Co., 1894).

14. W. A. Emboden, *Ritual Use of Cannabis Sativa L.: A historical ethnographic survey,* in P. T. Furst, ed., *Flesh of the Gods: The Ritual Use of Hallucinogens* (New York: Praeger, 1974).

15. Bennett et al., *Green Gold*, 37.

16. Baron Ernst von Bibra, *Plant Intoxicants* (Rochester, Vt.: Healing Arts Press, 1995), 161.

17. Bennett et al., *Green Gold*, 39–40.

18. Ibid., 46.

19. Ibid., 55.

20. Ibid., 62.

21. Ibid., 57.

22. Ibid., 85.

23. Ibid., 115.

24. William A. Emboden, Jr., *Narcotic Plants* (New York: Macmillan, 1972), 14.

25. Ibid.

26. Joseph Needham, *Science and Civilization* (Cambridge: Cambridge University Press, 1976).

27. Bennett et al., *Green Gold*, 126.

28. Luis Yanchi, *The Essential Book of Traditional Chinese Medicine*, vol. 2 (New York: Columbia University Press, 1988).

29. Bennett et al., *Green Gold*, 126.

30. Rebekah Mulvaney, *Rastafari and Reggae* (Westport, Conn.: Greenwood Press, 1990), 36.

31. Andrew Weil, *Health and Healing* (Boston: Houghton Mifflin, 1983), 222–223.

32. Mircea Eliade, *Patanjali and Yoga* (New York: Shocken, 1969), 179.

33. Harry Avis, *Drugs and Life* (Dubuque, Iowa: Wm. C. Brown, 1990), 38.

34. McKenna, "Plan, Plant, Planet," 5.

35. Ibid., 7.

36. Andrew Weil, *Chocolate to Morphine* (Boston: Houghton Mifflin, 1983), 25.

37. Bennett et al., *Green Gold*, 273fn.

38. Alfred Freedman et al., *Modern Synopsis of Comprehensive Textbook of Psychiatry II* (Baltimore: Williams & Wilkins, 1976), 667.

39. Robert De Ropp, *The Master Game* (New York: Delacorte, 1968), 43–44.

Notes to Chapter 4

1. Sources describing the evolution of cannabis hemp in central Asia include: Te-K'un Cheng, *Archaeology in China*, vol. 1 (Cambridge: W. Fleffer & Son, 1959); Hui-Lin Li, "The Origin and Use of Cannabis in Eastern Asia," *Economic Botany* 28 (July–September 1974): 293–301; J. G. Anderson, *Bulletin of the Geographical Society of China* 5 (1923): 26; Kwang-chih Chang, *The Archaeology of Ancient China* (New Haven, Conn.: Yale University Press, 1986); K'ao-Ku, *Archaeology* 7 (1984): 654–663; and *Chinese Archaeological Abstracts* 6 (1978): 498.

2. Joseph Needham, *Science and Civilization* (Cambridge University Press, 1976).

3. M. D. Merlin, *Man and Marijuana* (Rutherford, N.J.: Fairleigh Dickenson University Press, 1968).

4. Hui-Lin Li, "An Archaeological and Historical Account of Cannabis in China," *Economic Botany* 28 (October–December 1974): 437–448.

5. Cho-yun Hsu, *Han Agriculture* (Seattle, Wash.: University of Washington Press, 1980), 70–71, 81, 82–83, 226, 262, 280, 282, 287, 289, 309.

6. Sources describing the invention of vegetable-fiber paper include: Pan Jixing, *Wenwu* 9 (1973); 45–51, and Abel, *Marihuana: The First Twelve Thousand Years.*

7. Hsu, *Han Agriculture*, 282, 283, 287.

8. Sources describing the use of hemp in Chinese medicine include: Dominique Hoizey and Marie-J. Hoizey, *A History of Chinese Medicine* (Vancouver, B.C.: University of British Columbia Press, 1993); Lui Yanchi, *The Essential Book of Traditional Chinese Medicine*, vol. 2 (New York: Columbia University Press, 1988).

9. *Chinese Archaeological Abstracts* 6 (1978): 252.

10. Edward Schafer, *The Golden Peaches of Samarkand* (Berkeley, Calif.: University of California Press, 1963), 195.

11. Conrad, *Hemp: Lifeline to the Future,* 19.

12. R. Chopra and I. Chopra, *Chopra's Indigenous Drugs of India* (Calcutta: U. N. Dhur & Sons, 1958).

13. Abel, *Marihuana: The First Twelve Thousand Years,* 24.

14. Richard Burton, *The Thousand and One Nights* (New York: Modern Library, 1932).

15. J. C. Mardrus and P. Mathers, *The Thousand and One Nights*, vol. 3 (New York: Routledge, 1989), 520–523.

16. Abel, *Marihuana: The First Twelve Thousand Years,* 43–57.

17. Lise Manniche, *An Ancient Egyptian Herbal* (Austin, Texas: University of Texas Press, 1989).

18. Honor Frost, *Natural History* 96, no. 12 (December 1987): 58–67.

19. Abel, *Marihuana: The First Twelve Thousand Years,* 38–39.

20. Ibid., 39.

21. Ibid., 41–43.

22. Peter T. Furst, *Flesh of the Gods* (Prospect Heights, Il.: Waveland Press, 1972), 227.

23. M. Levey and N. Al-Khaledy, *The Medical Formulary of Al-Samarqandi* (Philadelphia: University of Pennsylvania Press, 1967).

24. N. J. Van Der Merwe, "Cannabis Smoking in 13th- and 14th-Century Ethiopia," in *Cannabis and Culture,* ed. V. Rubin (The Hague: Mouton, 1975).

25. A. T. Bryant, *The Zulu People* (New York: Negro Universities Press, 1970).

26. Timothy Painne, *An Abstract of . . . A Treatise on Hemp* (Boston: Edes and Gill, 1766).

27. T. Frank, *An Economic Survey of Ancient Rome* (Patterson, N.J.: Pageant Books, 1959), 131, 616, 823–824.

28. Peter Laven, *Renaissance Italy, 1464–1534* (New York: G. P. Putnam & Sons, 1966), 18, 21, 27, 31, 39, 47.

29. The Wilmersdorf tomb is discussed in: W. Reininger, "Remnants from Prehistoric Times," in G. Andrews and J. Vinkenoog, *The Book of Grass* (New York: Grove Press, 1967), 14; and J. Werner, *Antiquity* 38 (1964): 201–216.

30. Sir James G. Frazer, *Balder The Beautiful* (New York: Macmillan, 1935).

31. Abel, *Marihuana: The First Twelve Thousand Years,* 67–68.

32. Francois Rabelais, *Gargantua and Pantagruel,* trans. Burton Raffel (New York: W. W. Norton, 1990).

33. Fernand Braudel, *The Mediterranean and the Mediterranean World in the Age of Phillip II* (New York: Harper & Row, 1973), 430, 611, 779, 1225.

34. Abel, *Marihuana: The First Twelve Thousand Years,* 148–149.

35. Baron Ernst von Bibra, *Plant Intoxicants,* 147.

36. Alfred W. Crosby, *America, Russia, Hemp, and Napoléon* (Ohio State University Press, 1965).

37. H. Godwin, *Antiquity* 41 (1967): 42–49.

38. J. Grattan and C. Singer, *Anglo-Saxon Magic and Medicine* (London: Folcroft Library Editions, 1971), 123.

39. A. De Pasquale, *Estratto dai Lavori dell'Instituto di Farmacognosia dell'Universita di Messina* 5 (1967): 24; and P. Kemp, *The Healing Ritual* (London: Faber & Faber, 1935), 57, 198.

40. A. V. De Espinoza, *Description of the Indies* (Washington, DC: Smithsonian Institute Press, 1960), 453, 728.

41. E. Lipson, *The Economic History of England* (London: A. & C. Black, 1931), 2: 109, 187, 227, 319, 351; 3: 21, 182–185, 206, 354, 407, 429, 471, 477.

42. T. Tusser, *Five Hundred Points of Good Husbandrie* (London: n.p., 1580).

43. Joan Thirsk and J. P. Cooper, *Seventeenth Century Economic Documents* (Oxford: Clarendon Press, 1972), 110.

44. W. Cunningham, *The Growth of English Industry and Commerce* (New York: Augustus M. Kelley, 1968).

45. Joan Thirsk and J. P. Cooper, *Seventeenth-Century Economic Documents,* 154.

46. Ibid., 738.

47. Abel, *Marihuana: The First Twelve Thousand Years,* 73–75.

Notes to Chapter 5

1. Cyrus Gordon, *Before Columbus: Links Between the Old World and Ancient America* (New York: Crown Books, 1971), 46–49, 170–177; Henriette Mertz, *Pale Ink: Two Ancient Records of Chinese Explorations in America* (1953; reprint, Chicago: Swallow Press, 1972).

2. W. H. Holmes, *Prehistoric Textile Art of Eastern United States, 13th Annual Report* (Washington, DC: Smithsonian Institution Bureau of Ethnology, 1891–1892).

3. Richard Hakluyt, *The English Voyages*, vol. 8 (Glasgow: n.p., 1903), 268, 353, 429.

4. T. B. Costain, *The White and the Gold* (New York: Doubleday, 1954); John Swanton, *The Indians of the Southeastern United States*, Smithsonian Bulletin no. 137 (New York: Greenwood Press, 1969), 306.

5. Frances Little, *Early American Textiles* (New York: Century Co., 1931), 14.

6. Antoine Le Page du Pratz, *History of Louisiana* (Paris, 1758; reprint, Baton Rouge, La.: Claitor's, 1972), 238.

7. Robert Bell, ed., *Select Essays on Raising and Dressing Flax and Hemp* (Philadelphia: Robert Bell, publisher, 1777).

8. L. Morton, *Robert Carter of Nomini Hall* (Williamsburg, Va.: Colonial Williamsburg, Inc., 1941), 156.

9. Thomas Paine, *Common Sense,* 1776.

10. All excerpts from *The Diaries of George Washington* (Boston: Houghton-Mifflin, 1925).

11. Robert C. Baron, *The Garden and Farm Books of Thomas Jefferson* (Golden, Colo.: Fulcrum, Inc., 1987).

12. William Hutchinson and William M. Rachal, *The Papers of James Madison* (Chicago: University of Chicago Press, 1963), vol. 3: 114, 126; vol. 4: 29; vol. 5: 183; vol. 7: 84, 170, 361.

13. E. M. Betts, *Thomas Jefferson's Farm Book* (Princeton, N.J.: Princeton University Press, 1953), 252.

14. Edwin T. Martin, *Thomas Jefferson: Scientist* (New York: Collier Books, 1961), 88–90.

15. Alfred W. Crosby, Jr., *America, Russia, Hemp and Napolean* (Columbus, Ohio: Ohio State University Press; 1965).

16. Edward M. Brecher, *Licit and Illicit Drugs* (Boston: Little, Brown, 1972), 404, 409.

17. "Pot and Presidents," *Green Egg* (21 June 1975).

18. Brent Moore, *The Hemp Industry in Kentucky* (Lexington, Ky.: Press

of James Hughes, 1905), 13–14.

19. C. P. Nettels, *The Emergence of a National Economy* (New York: Holt, Reinhart & Winston, 1962), vol. 2: 110, 171; vol. 3, 15, 116, 117, 326, 327.

20. Conrad, *Hemp: Lifeline to the Future,* 40.

Notes to Chapter 6

1. Fitz H. Ludlow, *The Hasheesh Eater: Being Passages from the Life of a Pythagorean* (New York: Harper & Bros., 1857).

2. Abel, *Marihuana: The First Twelve Thousand Years,* 178.

3. Daniel Shealy et al., eds. *Louisa May Alcott: Selected Fiction* (Boston: Little, Brown & Co., 1990), 117–127.

4. David F. Musto, *The American Disease* (New Haven, Conn.: Yale University Press, 1973), 217; and John Helmer, *Drugs and Minority Oppression* (New York: Seabury Press, 1975), 67.

5. Conrad, *Hemp: Lifeline to the Future,* 43.

6. A. E. Fossier, *New Orleans Medical and Surgical Journal* 44 (1931): 247–250.

7. *International Medical Digest* 77 (1937): 183–187.

8. Larry Sloman, *Reefer Madness: The History of Marijuana in America.*

9. Herer, *The Emperor Wears No Clothes,* 27.

10. M. Mezzrow and B. Wolfe: *Really the Blues* (New York: Random House, 1946).

11. Herer, *The Emperor Wears No Clothes,* 24–27.

12. R. F. Smith, *Report of Investigation in the State of Texas, Particularly Along the Mexican Border, of the Traffic in, and Consumption of the Drug Generally Known as 'Indian Hemp' or Cannabis indica* (U.S. Dept. of Agriculture, 1917).

13. U.S. Treasury Department, Bureau of Narcotics, *Traffic in Opium and Other Dangerous Drugs for the Year Ended, December 31, 1931* (Washington, DC: Government Printing Office, 1932).

14. Conrad, *Hemp: Lifeline to the Future,* 45.

15. H. J. Anslinger and Courtney R. Cooper, *American Magazine* 124 (July 1937): 19, 150.

16. Richard Bonnie and Charles Whitebread, *The Marihuana Conviction* (Charlottesville, Va.: University of Virginia Press, 1974).

17. H. J. Anslinger and Will Ousler, *The Murderers* (New York: Farrar, Straus, & Cudahy, 1961), 35–36; and C. R. Cooper, *Here's to Crime* (Boston: Little Brown, 1937), 333–338.

18. Musto, *The American Disease,* 224–227.

19. All quotations from the Ways and Means Committee in U.S. Congress, Committee on Ways and Means, House of Representatives, 75th Congress, 1st session (April 27–30, May 4, 1937), on HR 6385.

20. *Rolling Stone,* August 1983.

21. U.S. Congress, House of Representatives, *Congressional Record,*

75th Congress, 1st session (1937), 5575.

22. U.S. Congress, Senate Committee on Finance, 1st Session (1937).

Notes to Chapter 7

1. *Hemp for Victory,* distributed by Help Eliminate Marijuana Prohibition, 5632 Van Nuys #210, Van Nuys, CA 91401.

2. Sackett and Hobbs: *Hemp: A War Crop* (New York: Mason & Hanger, 1942).

3. Kefauver Committee Hearings, Part 14, 119.

4. *Congressional Record,* 97th congress, 1951.

5. U.N. Single Convention on Narcotic Drugs, 1961, Article 28(3).

6. Proceedings: White House Conference on Narcotic and Drug Abuse (Sept. 27–28, 1962) (Washington, DC: Government Printing Office, 1963).

8. *Washington Post* (24 February 1970): D-1, col. 3.

9. John Steinbeck IV, *In Touch* (New York, 1969), 97.

10. William Novak, *High Culture* (Boston: CIA Publications, 1980).

11. Richard C. Schroeder, *The Politics of Drugs: An American Dilemma* (Washington, DC: Congressional Quarterly, 1980).

12. Edward Jay Epstein, *Agency of Fear: Opiates and Political Power in America* (New York: Putnam, 1977).

13. P. Landrigan et al., *American Jour-*

nal of Public Health 73, no. 7 (July 1983): 784–788.

14. Herer, *The Emperor Wears No Clothes,* 86–87.

15. Ibid.

16. NewsBank XV (1984): INT 63: C14.

17. NewsBank XXI (1990): LAW 82: F3.

18. NewsBank XVII (1986): LAW 91: D3.

19. John Ensslin, "Boy Spots Marijuana in House, Turns in His Parents," *Rocky Mountain News* (CO), (24 Sept. 1991); NewsBank XXIII (1992): HEALTH 110: G6; ibid., (1992): LAW 12: E13.

20. NewsBank XIX (1988): LAW 106: D13.

21. NewsBank XIX (1988): LAW 106: F4.

22. NewsBank XIX (1988): LAW 106: F7.

23. NewsBank XXIV (1993): LAW 56: F2.

24. NewsBank XXII (1991) LAW 40: D12; ibid., (1991) LAW 81: D1.

25. *Boston Globe,* Special Report: Overdosing on the Drug War, (24–27 September 1995).

26. Ibid.

27. Eric Schlosser, "Reefer Madness," *Atlantic Monthly* (August 1994): 45.

28. Schlosser, "Marijuana and the Law," Atlantic Monthly (September 1994): 89.

29. Schlosser, "Reefer Madness," 55.

30. NewsBank XXIII (1992): LAW 12: A13, San Diego, California, *Union* (12 February 1992); and NewsBank XXI (1990): LAW 57: D9.

31. NewsBank XXI (1990): LAW 40; C14, and NewsBank XXIV (1993): LAW 56: E9.

32. NewsBank XXII (1991): LAW 40: A9.

33. Mark Curriden, "Rising Use of Police 'Snitches' Questioned" *Atlanta Journal* (31 March 1991).

34. NewsBank XXIV (1993): LAW 17: A6.

35. *Journal of the International Hemp Association* 2, Vol.1 (1995).

36. Lester Grinspoon and James B. Bakalar, *Marihuana, the Forbidden Medicine* (New Haven, Conn.: Yale University Press, 1993).

37. Press Review of Drug Related Articles, Baltimore Newspapers (*Sun* and *News American*): Mayor's Office of Drug Abuse Control, Baltimore, 1973).

38. Robert C. Randall, ed., *Marijuana, Medicine, & the Law* (Washington, DC: Galen Press, 1988).

39. Ibid.

40. Robert Saveland and Bray, *American Trends in Cannabis Use Among States With Different and Changing Legal Regimes* (Ottawa: Bureau of Tobacco Control and Biometrics, Health and Welfare, 1980); NewsBank XIV (1983): LAW 67: D5; Eric Single, *The Impact of Marijuana Decriminalization in Research Advances in Alcohol & Drug Problems* (Addiction Research Foundation/Plenum Press, 1981), 423; Robert Bomboy, Major Newspaper Coverage of Drug Issues, April 1974, Drug Abuse Council.

41. *The Drug Policy Letter,* 24 (Fall 1994), 22.

42. The drug policy debate is carried out in sources including: Arnold S. Trebach, *Justice Quarterly* I (1984): 125–144; and *The Great Drug War: Radical Proposals That Could Make America Safe Again* (New York: Macmillan, 1987); Bruce K. Alexander, *Peaceful Measures: Canada's Way Out of the War on Drugs* (Toronto: University of Toronto Press, 1990); R. Bayer and G. Oppenheimer, eds., *Confronting Drug Policy* (Cambridge: Cambridge University Press, 1993); David Boaz, ed., *Crisis in Drug Prohibition* (Washington, DC: Cato Institute, 1990); John Helmer, *Drugs and Minority Oppression* (New York: Seabury Press, 1975); John Kaplan, *Marijuana: The New Prohibition* (New York: World Publishing Co./Pocket Books, 1970); Mark A. Kleiman, *Marijuana: Costs of Abuse, Costs of Control* (Westport, Conn.: Greenwood Press, 1989); Melvyn B. Krauss and Edward P. Lazear, *Searching for Alternatives: Drug-Control Policy in the United States* (Stanford, Calif.: Hoover Institution Press, 1991); David F. Musto, *The American Disease: Origins of Narcotic Control* (New Haven, Conn.: Yale University Press, 1973); Richard C. Schroeder, *The Politics of Drugs: An American Dilemma* (Washington DC: Congressional Quarterly, Inc., 1980); and Steven Wisotsy, *Beyond the War on Drugs: Overcoming a Failed Public Policy* (New York: Prometheus Books, 1990).

43. NewsBank XXIV (1993): LAW 77: C6; and NewsBank XVI (1985): LAW 42: E2.

44. The Canadian Government Commission of Inquiry, The Non-Medical Use of Drugs: *Interim Report* (Baltimore, Md.: Penguin Books, 1970); and *Cannabis: A Report of the Commission of Inquiry into the Non-Medical Use of Drugs* (Ottawa: Information Canada, 1972).

45. Anderson, Patrick, *High in America* (New York: Viking Press, 1981); and NewsBank XXI (1990): LAW 36: A6.

46. NewsBank XXII (1991): HEALTH 123: A9, XXIII (1992): HEALTH 28: E12, and XXIII (1992): HEALTH 114: D12; J. J. Kettenes-Van Den Bosch et al., *J. Ethnopharmacology* 2 (1980): 197-231; *Federal Register* 37 (1 September 1972): 18093; and NewsBank XXII (1991): HEALTH 123: A12.

47. *Federal Register* 54 (249) (29 December 1988): 53784; and R. C. Randall, ed., *Marijuana, Medicine, & The Law.*

48. NewsBank XXII (1991) LAW 40: C10, D12.

49. NewsBank XIX (1988): LAW 106: B9; ibid., LAW 107: D2.

50. NewsBank XXI (1990): LAW 82: D13.

51. Kurt L. Schmoke, *American Behavioral Scientist* 32 (January–February 1989): 231–232.

52. *San Francisco Examiner* (22 August 1993).

53. NewsBank XXV (1994): LAW 39: D2.

54. NewsBank XXV (1994): LAW 39: D4.

55. *The Drug Policy Letter* 23, (July/August 1994), 16.

56. A. C. M. Jansen, *Cannabis In Amsterdam* (Muiderberg: D. Coutinho, 1991).

57. *Marijuana: A Signal of Misunderstanding,* (New York: New American Library, 1972).

58. Vera Rubin and L. Comitas, *Ganja in Jamaica: A Medical Anthropological Study of Chronic Marijuana Use* (The Hague: Mouton & Co., 1975).

BIBLIOGRAPHY

Abel, Ernest L. *A Comprehensive Guide to the Cannabis Literature.* Westwood, Conn.: Greenwood Press, 1979.

———. *Marihuana: The First Twelve Thousand Years.* New York: Plenum Press, 1980.

———. *A Marihuana Dictionary.* Westwood, Conn.: Greenwood Press, 1982.

Alexander, Bruce K. *Peaceful Measures: Canada's Way Out of the 'War on Drugs'.* Toronto: University of Toronto Press, 1990.

Allen, James L. *The Reign of Law. A Tale of the Kentucky Hemp Fields.* New York: MacMillan Co., 1900.

Anderson, Patrick. *High in America.* New York: Viking Press, 1981.

Andrews, George, and Simon Vinkenoog, eds. *The Book of Grass: An Anthology of Indian Hemp.* New York: Grove Press, Inc., 1967.

Bayer, R., and G. Oppenheimer, eds. *Confronting Drug Policy.* Cambridge: Cambridge University Press, 1993.

Bennett, Chris, Lynn Osburn, and Judy Osburn. *Green Gold, the Tree of Life: Marijuana in Magic and Religion.* Frazier Park, Calif.: Access Unlimited, 1995.

Boaz, David, ed. *The Crisis in Drug Prohibition.* Washington, DC: Cato Institute, 1990.

Boire, Richard Glen. *Marijuana Law.* Berkeley, Calif.: Ronin Publishing, 1993.

Bonnie, Richard J., and Charles H. Whitebread. *The Marihuana Conviction: A History of Marihuana Prohibition in the United States.* Charlottesville, Va.: University Press of Virginia, 1974.

Braude, M. C., and S. Szara, eds. *Pharmacology of Marihuana*. New York: Raven Press, 1976.

Clarke, Robert C. *Marijuana Botany*. Berkeley, Calif.: And/Or Press, 1981.

Cohen, S., and R. C. Stillman, eds. *The Therapeutic Potential of Marihuana*. New York: Plenum Medical Book Co., 1976.

Conrad, Chris. *Hemp: Lifeline to the Future*. Los Angeles, Calif.: Creative Xpressions Publications, 1993.

Crosby, Alfred W. *America, Russia, Hemp, and Napoleon*. Columbus, Ohio: Ohio State University Press, 1965.

Drake, W. D., Jr. *Marijuana: The Cultivators' Handbook*. Berkeley, Calif.: Wingbow Press, 1979.

Frank, M., and E. Rosenthal. *Marijuana Grower's Guide*. Berkeley, Calif.: And/Or Press, 1978.

Frazier, Jack. *The Marijuana Farmers*. New Orleans: Solar Age Press, 1972.

———. *The Great American Hemp Industry*. Peterstown, W.Va.: Solar Age Press, 1991.

Grinspoon, Lester. *Marihuana Reconsidered*. Cambridge, Mass.: Harvard University Press, 1971.

Grinspoon, L., and James Bakalar. *Marihuana, the Forbidden Medicine*. New Haven, Conn.: Yale University Press, 1993.

Hawken, Paul. *The Ecology of Commerce*. New York: HarperCollins, 1993.

Helmer, John. *Drugs and Minority Oppression*. New York: Seabury Press, 1975.

Hendin, Herbert, et al. *Living High: Daily Marijuana Use Among Adults*. New York: Human Sciences Press, 1987.

Herer, Jack. *The Emperor Wears No Clothes*. Van Nuys, Calif.: Hemp Publishing, 1993.

Himmelstein, Jerome L. *The Strange Career of Marihuana*. Westport, Conn.: Greenwood Press, 1983.

Hopkins, J. F. *A History of the Hemp Industry in Kentucky*. Lexington, Ky.: University of Kentucky Press, 1951.

Hoye, David. *Cannabis Alchemy*. Berkeley, Calif.: And/Or Press, 1973.

Indian Hemp Drugs Commission. *Marijuana: Report of the Indian Hemp Drugs Commission, 1893–1894*. Silver Spring, Md.: T. Jefferson Publishing Co., 1969.

Jansen, A. C. M. *Cannabis In Amsterdam*. Muiderberg: Dick Coutinho, 1991.

Kaplan, John. *Marijuana: The New Prohibition*. New York: World Publishing Co./ Pocket Books, 1970.

Kleiman, Mark A. *Marijuana: Costs of Abuse, Costs of Control*. Westport, Conn.: Greenwood Press, 1989.

Krauss, Melvyn B., and Lazear, Edward P. *Searching for Alternatives: Drug-Control Policy in the United States*. Stanford, Calif.: Hoover Institution Press, 1991.

Lansky, Mitch. *Beyond the Beauty Strip*. Gardiner, Maine: Tilbury House, 1992.

THE GREAT BOOK OF HEMP

Ludlow, F. H. *The Hasheesh Eater: Being Passages from the Life of a Pythagorean.* New York: Harper & Bros., 1857.

Maykut, Madeleine. *Health Consequences of Acute and Chronic Marihuana Use.* New York: Pergamon Press, 1984.

Mayor's Committee on Marihuana. *The Marihuana Problem in the City of New York.* Lancaster, Pa.: J. Cattell Press, 1944; repr. Metuchen, N.J.: Scarecrow Reprint Corp., 1973.

Mechoulam, Raphael. *Marijuana: Chemistry, Pharmacology, Metabolism and Clinical Effects.* New York: Academic Press, 1973.

Mendelson, J. H., et al., eds. *The Use of Marijuana: A Psychological and Physiological Inquiry.* New York: Plenum Press, 1974.

Mikuriya, Todd H., ed. *Marijuana: Medical Papers 1839–1972.* Oakland, Calif.: Medi-Comp Press, 1973.

Miller, L. L., ed. *Marijuana: Effects on Human Behavior.* New York: Academic Press, 1974.

Miller, Carol, and Donald Wirtshafter. *The Hemp Seed Cookbook.* Athens, Ohio: The Ohio Hempery Inc., 1993.

Moore, Laurence A. *Marijuana (Cannabis) Bibliography, 1960–1968.* Los Angeles, Calif.: Bruin Humanist Forum, 1969.

Musto, David F. *The American Disease: Origins of Narcotic Control.* New Haven, Conn.: Yale University Press, 1973.

Nahas, G. G., and C. Latour, eds. *Cannabis Physiopathology, Epidemiology, Detection.* Boca Raton, Fla.: CRC Press, 1993.

Nahas, G. G., and W. Paton, eds. *Marihuana: Biological Effects.* Oxford: Pergamon Press, 1979.

Nahas, G. G., et al., eds. *Marihuana: Chemistry, Biochemistry, and Cellular Effects.* New York: Springer-Verlag, 1976.

Novak, William. *High Culture.* Boston: CIA Publications, 1980.

Paton, W. D. M., and J. Crown. *Cannabis and its Derivatives.* Oxford: Oxford University Press, 1972.

Relman, Arnold, ed. *Marijuana and Health.* Washington, DC: National Academy Press, 1982.

Roffman, Roger A. *Marijuana As Medicine.* Seattle: Madrona Publishers, 1982.

Rosenthal, Ed, ed. *Hemp Today.* Oakland, Calif.: Quick American Archives, 1994.

Roulac, John, ed. *Industrial Hemp.* Ojai, Calif.: HempTech, 1995.

Rubin, Vera, and L. Comitas. *Ganja in Jamaica: A Medical Anthropological Study of Chronic Marijuana Use.* The Hague: Mouton & Co., 1975.

Rubin, V., ed. *Cannabis and Culture.* The Hague: Mouton & Co., 1975.

Schroeder, Richard C. *The Politics of Drugs: An American Dilemma.* Washington, DC: Congressional Quarterly, Inc., 1980.

Sloman, Larry. *Reefer Madness: Marijuana in America.* New York: Bobbs-Merrill Co., 1979.

236

Solomon, David, ed. *The Marijuana Papers.* New York: Bobbs-Merrill Co., 1966.

Symons, A., trans. *Baudelaire: Prose and Poetry.* New York: Albert and Charles Boni, 1926.

Szasz, Thomas. *Ceremonial Chemistry: The Ritual Persecution of Drugs, Addicts, and Pushers.* New York: Anchor Press/Doubleday, 1974.

Tart, Charles. *On Being Stoned.* Palo Alto, Calif.: Science and Behavior Books, 1971.

Tinklenberg, J. R., ed. *Marijuana and Health Hazards: Methodological Issues in Current Research.* New York: Academic Press, Inc., 1975.

Trebach, Arnold, and James Inciardi. *Legalize It? Debating American Drug Policy.* Washington, DC: American University Press, 1993.

U.S. Commission on Marihuana and Drug Abuse. *Marihuana: Signal of Misunderstanding.* Washington, DC: U.S. Government Printing Office, 1972.

Van der Werf, Hayo. *Crop Physiology of Fibre Hemp* (Cannabis Sativa *L.*). Wageningen, the Netherlands: Wageningen Agricultural University, 1994.

von Bibra, Baron Ernst. *Plant Intoxicants.* Rochester, Vt.: Healing Arts Press, 1995.

Waller, Coy W., and Jacqueline Denny. *Annotated Bibliography of Marihuana. 1964–1970.* University, Miss.: University of Mississippi Press, 1971.

Weil, Andrew. *The Natural Mind.* Boston: Houghton Mifflin Co., 1972.

Weisheit, Ralph A. *Domestic Marijuana: A Neglected Industry.* Westport, Conn.: Greenwood Press, 1992.

Wirtshafter, Don, ed. *The Schlichten Papers.* Athens, Ohio: The Ohio Hempery, Inc., 1994.

Wisotsky, Steven. *Beyond the War on Drugs: Overcoming a Failed Public Policy.* New York: Prometheus Books, 1990.

Wolstenholme, G., et al., eds. *Hashish: Its Chemistry and Pharmacology.* CIBA Foundation Study Group 21, 1965.

INDEX

A Note on Hemp Paper

Every reasonable effort was made by Inner Traditions to print *The Great Book of Hemp* on hemp paper. Unfortunately, imported hemp paper is still very expensive for large-scale use, and we were unable to do so. What must happen to make hemp paper affordable for all applications? *Demand.* As demand for hemp continues to skyrocket, hemp prices will continue to fall. Most importantly, we urge you, the reader, to demand that hemp be allowed to grow again on the nation's farms. And we at Inner Traditions promise to make the next edition of *The Great Book of Hemp* a tree-free book.